THE HUNGER CODE

JASON FUNG, MD

THE HUNGER CODE

RESETTING YOUR
BODY'S FAT THERMOSTAT
IN THE AGE OF
ULTRA-PROCESSED FOOD

GREYSTONE BOOKS

Vancouver/Berkeley/London

Greystone Books Ltd.
greystonebooks.com

Cataloguing data available from Library and Archives Canada
ISBN 978-1-77840-156-5 (cloth)
ISBN 978-1-77840-157-2 (epub)

Editing by Lucy Kenward
Copyediting by Lenore Hietkamp
Proofreading by Alison Strobel
Indexing by Stephen Ullstrom
Jacket design by DSGN Dept.
Text design by Fiona Siu

Printed and bound in Canada on FSC® certified paper at Friesens. The FSC® label
means that materials used for the product have been responsibly sourced.

Greystone Books thanks the Canada Council for the Arts, the British Columbia Arts
Council, the Province of British Columbia through the Book Publishing Tax Credit,
and the Government of Canada for supporting our publishing activities.

EU Safety Information: Easy Access System Europe, Mustamäe tee 50,
10621 Tallinn, Estonia, gpsr.requests@easproject.com.

Canada

BRITISH COLUMBIA

BRITISH COLUMBIA ARTS COUNCIL
An agency of the Province of British Columbia

CERTIFIED CANADIAN PUBLISHER

Canada Council for the Arts   Conseil des arts du Canada

MIX
Paper | Supporting responsible forestry
FSC
www.fsc.org   FSC® C016245

Greystone Books gratefully acknowledges the xʷməθkʷəy̓əm (Musqueam),
Sḵwx̱wú7mesh (Squamish), and səlilwətaɫ (Tsleil-Waututh) peoples on
whose land our Vancouver head office is located.

Dedicated to my parents, Mui Hun and Wing Fung,
Michael and Margaret Chan, who have always supported me.
Their watch has never ended.

Also dedicated to my wife, Mina, who inspires me daily,
and my boys, Jonathan and Matthew, for their boundless energy.

CONTENTS

Part 4: How to Manage Hunger

PREFACE

T HE FIRST STEP to solving a problem is to admit that one exists.

I once attended a department meeting where the director discussed the accomplishments of the hospital's center for integrative medicine. Since the center opened to great fanfare several years earlier, this department of five people had done one workplace survey and taken over the lead on a program where student volunteers gave free massages to patients and staff.

"Wow," I thought. "That's *it*? That really sucks." I could have done that work myself in about two days. But I didn't say anything because it wasn't really my business. And as the director sat down, other people commented, "Congratulations, this is very exciting" and "Excellent work."

The hospital had obviously pissed away all the money it had raised for the center, but we needed to pretend that all was great. Nobody wanted to yell: "The emperor has no clothes!" This delusion is generally how any bureaucracy works. Rather than acknowledging the truth, we pretend that everything is super awesome, thank you very much. Good job, everybody, good job.

This scenario is not unique to my hospital; it is pervasive in all of public health. We pretend that we (the academic research community, doctors, dietitians, the nutritional authorities) are doing great work, even as a tidal wave of obesity and type 2 diabetes that dwarfs anything the world has ever seen destroys us. Nobody wants to admit there is a problem—and therefore we have not taken the first steps toward solving it.

It is obvious that things are not going well. You can look at any statistic about global obesity and it will be bad. Horrible, actually. In 1985, the prevalence of obesity did not exceed 10 percent in any state in the United States of America. By 2024, not a single state managed to keep their prevalence of obesity below 20 percent, and only three lonely states fell below 25 percent.[1] Oh my. Nobody *wants* to be overweight or obese, so what's the disconnect?

The dominant view since the 1970s has been that "Eating too many calories" causes obesity, and therefore the solution is "Eating fewer calories." I learned this idea growing up in the 1970s, again during medical school in the 1990s, and I hear it still today. You've probably heard the "Calories In, Calories Out" phrase a million times. This calorie-centric view of obesity as an energy balance problem goes something like this:

1. You eat more calories than you burn.
2. Excess calories are stored as body fat.
3. The solution, therefore, is to eat fewer calories or exercise more to burn more calories.

Does this universally accepted weight-loss advice work? Not even a little. Logically, if certain advice is not working, then we should change it. *But* that also means we must admit there is a problem. And no bureaucracy ever admits that a problem exists.

The obsessive focus on calories is neither useful nor effective. Since the 1970s, we have been getting heavier and heavier. Why keep giving the same tired advice and hoping for different results? That is literally the definition of insanity. Let's face that hard truth and start moving forward.

Percentage of American adults with BMI >30
(percentage of Americans who have obesity)[2]

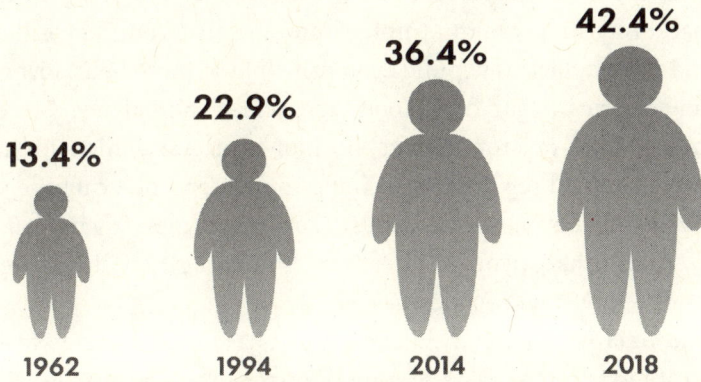

13.4% **22.9%** **36.4%** **42.4%**

1962   1994   2014   2018

"Expert" advice:

Eat fewer
calories!

Eat fewer
calories!

Eat fewer
calories!

Eat fewer
calories!

Time to think differently?

THIS IS *NOT* A DIET BOOK

THE SECOND STEP to solving a problem is to follow good advice.

We have a magic formula for everything. For example, when putting together a boy band, you need the tough guy, the fun guy, the sensitive guy, the nice guy, and the jock. Mix in some rudimentary dance steps and a catchy pop tune, and magic happens. Diet books also follow a winning formula. I will reveal the secrets, right here, right now, for free!

1. **The Promise:** Plain old, boring weight loss isn't enough anymore. You must promise more, more, more! "Effortless" weight loss. Without sacrifice. Without hunger. While still eating cookies. "Rapid" weight loss. It doesn't really matter whether these promises are true or not, as long as they sound good and are not completely impossible.

You can also throw in other promises. Your skin will clear up. Your asthma will go away. Your wrinkles will disappear. Dogs will love you. You'll be a *Jeopardy!* master. You'll live to 100 or your money back! Anything you can think of, promise that your diet will do it.

2. **The Hook:** Pick any foundation principle or ingredient: low carbs, low calories, sugar-free, blood type, acid-alkali balance, Glycemic Index, Zone macronutrients, hormones, exercise, high-intensity exercise, meal replacements, grapefruit, green juice, cabbage soup. Make sure it is unexpected, unusual, and not completely implausible.

   Claim that if you do or eat this (one thing), you'll lose weight effortlessly and keep it off!

3. **The Secret:** Explain the diet trick that has remained undiscovered for the last 5000 years of human history, the one that magically targets fat cells. For example, humans may have been growing and drinking coffee for many thousands of years, but what if they had crushed the green beans and eaten them instead! What if people had thought to juice their celery! Do Zone 2 exercise! Make cabbage soup!

   You can also claim that somebody is actively suppressing this secret. Do these headlines sound familiar? "The Fat Burning Secret *They* Don't Want You to Know!" "Belly-Busting Secrets of the Rich and Famous!"

4. **The Science:** Now, establish some science, or at least some pseudo-science. Meat is bad for you. Plants are bad for you. Fat is bad for you. Carbs are bad for you. Protein is bad for you. The sun is bad for you. Ancient aliens are behind the obesity epidemic.

5. **The Success Stories:** People love a good story, so pair a few before-and-after photos with one or more stories of transformation. For example: "I used to weigh 400 pounds and my hair was awful! Then I started juicing baby kale and, *ba-bam*, the weight melted right off! Plus, check out my soft, silky hair."

6. **The Plan—Phases I, II, and III with recipes:** Finally, provide the super-secret plan in three phases: the induction phase, the continuation phase, and the maintenance phase. Begin with some kind of severe restriction, then slowly reduce it over time. Add a

few recipes to make the plan easy to follow. Lamb's brain stew? Tree bark jerky?

There you have it: the winning formula you need to write a bestselling diet book. So how does *The Hunger Code* stack up?

1. The promise? No. *The Hunger Code* promises nothing but a deep scientific discussion about the causes of weight gain and weight loss.
2. The hook? No.
3. The secret? No.
4. The science? Yay. The whole book is about science, after all.
5. The success stories? Lots, but none of the my-life-transformed-in-twenty-four-hours variety.
6. The plan? No.
7. Recipes? That's a different book.

The final tally is 1/7, or a final grade of F. *The Hunger Code* is not a diet book. That's good. I didn't intend to write a diet book. Instead, I give dietary advice that is generations old: eat fewer ultra-processed foods, fast intermittently, and create the social bonds that will ensure success. That's *not* the latest and greatest advice. It's the tried and true.

In the decade since I wrote *The Obesity Code,* many people have benefited from learning that managing weight isn't about eating less and moving more but about what you eat and when you eat it. For people who have become insulin resistant and need to regulate their blood sugar quickly, a low-carbohydrate, high healthy fat diet and intermittent fasting can help reduce weight and reverse metabolic diseases. Yet as helpful as that advice is for many people, keeping the weight off long term can be a struggle. And that's where this book comes in. I consider it Part 2 of *The Obesity Code.*

In *The Hunger Code,* we move from the discussion of insulin and cortisol in *The Obesity Code* to consider the body fat thermostat more fully, along with recent information about how ultra-processed foods, food addictions, and the emotional and social aspects of obesity contribute to weight. This book explores the concept of hunger more fully, including homeostatic, hedonic, and conditioned hunger.

Why does this matter? Like everything else in life, if you know better, you can do better. Understanding what causes weight gain allows us to understand how to lose excess weight and, equally important, how to keep it off. The reason we eat is because we are hungry. Some of that hunger is physical, but as we'll see, a lot of that hunger is emotional and social too. *The Hunger Code* looks at the roots of our hunger and proposes real solutions. It is a book for anyone who struggles with their weight and for everyone who wants to eat healthier and live well.

THE QUICK START GUIDE

TODAY WE ARE overwhelmed with information but underwhelmed with understanding. This quick guide is a road map of the upcoming journey, or what my kids would call the tl;dr (too long; didn't read) summary. If you remember nothing else from reading this book, remember the three Golden Rules of weight loss:

1. Avoid ultra-processed foods.
2. Don't eat all the time. Fast regularly.
3. Commit to a health mindset and healthy social habits.

The Golden Rules address the root causes of all types of hunger and, together, they will allow you to achieve and maintain a healthy weight.

THE SCIENCE OF WEIGHT LOSS

THE STANDARD CONCEPT is that weight gain is a simple problem of Calories In, Calories Out. Eating too many calories causes you to gain body fat, and therefore weight loss is simply a matter of eating fewer calories, as this diagram appears to illustrate.

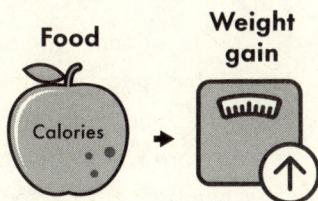

This simplistic perspective is known to be incomplete and mostly wrong, confirmed by decades of scientific evidence. The corollary to Calories In, Calories Out is Eat Less, Move More. Again, this advice is based on a largely incorrect understanding of human physiology and is therefore largely ineffective for losing weight.

The more accurate, physiological model recognizes that how much body fat we carry is dictated, like almost everything else about the human body, by changes in hormones. Some hormones increase body fat storage and some hormones decrease it. The body regulates the balance of these hormones using a homeostatic mechanism that's much like a body fat thermostat.

The foods that we eat influence which hormones our body produces. Food contains both

1. energy (calories) and
2. information (the body's hormonal response to the food).

Both are important. When we eat different foods, our body responds by releasing different hormones. For example, eating 200 calories of cookies releases the hormone insulin, which tells our body to store the incoming calories as fat. Little of the hormone that tells our body to feel full—glucagon-like peptide 1 (GLP-1)—is released. If we eat 200 calories of eggs, we don't release much insulin, so most of the calories are available as energy for the body. We release more GLP-1, which tells us to stop eating when we're full. The difference between these two is not the calories but the body's hormonal response, and that matters a lot.

This reality does not break any laws of thermodynamics; it simply means that some foods are more filling than other foods. It also means that some foods are more fattening than other foods. Steak is more filling than brownies. Cookies are more fattening than eggs.

When we eat these foods, the nutrients must be digested and then absorbed in the body. Many factors—including the structure of the food; the order in which foods are eaten; the timing of meals; the ways the foods are prepared, such as blending, cooking, and grinding—affect how quickly we digest and absorb the foods. The speed of digestion and absorption influences the hormonal effect and therefore affects weight gain.

Weight gain or loss results from whether we store or use the food energy we eat. The following diagram illustrates all the factors that contribute to weight. We will delve into each of these factors in more detail in Part 1.

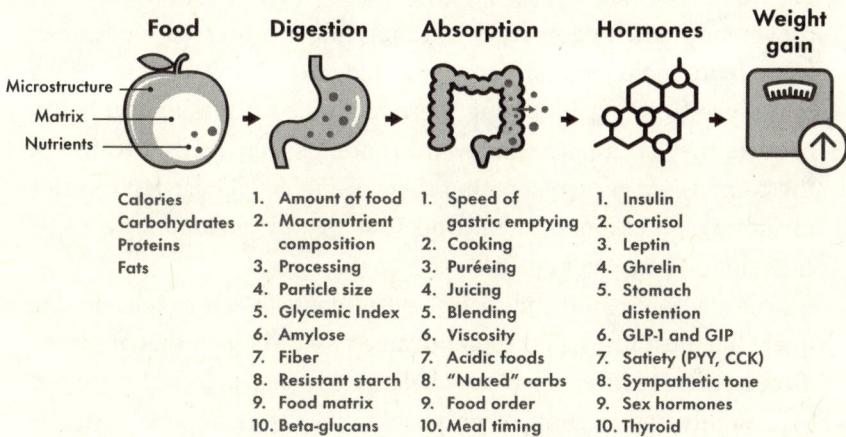

Food	Digestion	Absorption	Hormones	Weight gain
Microstructure Matrix Nutrients				
Calories Carbohydrates Proteins Fats	1. Amount of food 2. Macronutrient composition 3. Processing 4. Particle size 5. Glycemic Index 6. Amylose 7. Fiber 8. Resistant starch 9. Food matrix 10. Beta-glucans	1. Speed of gastric emptying 2. Cooking 3. Puréeing 4. Juicing 5. Blending 6. Viscosity 7. Acidic foods 8. "Naked" carbs 9. Food order 10. Meal timing	1. Insulin 2. Cortisol 3. Leptin 4. Ghrelin 5. Stomach distention 6. GLP-1 and GIP 7. Satiety (PYY, CCK) 8. Sympathetic tone 9. Sex hormones 10. Thyroid	

THE REALITY OF EATING BEHAVIOR

WHY DO WE EAT? Because we are hungry. We do we stop eating? Because we are full. Control the hunger, not the calories. The problem of "overeating" is really a problem of "over-hunger."

We have different types of hunger. The physical hunger that we experience as our body tries to get nutrients is **homeostatic hunger**. However, we eat for reasons other than nutrition. We also eat for pleasure or comfort, and that's **hedonic hunger**. And we eat out of habit, which is **conditioned hunger**. The three main types of hunger to manage are:

1. Homeostatic hunger (physical)
2. Hedonic hunger (emotional)
3. Conditioned hunger (environmental and social)

The science of weight loss is intimately linked to the psychology of eating behavior. Weight loss is about not just dietary change but behavior change. To succeed, we must address the physical, emotional, and social hungers that drive those behaviors.

The modern diet dominated by ultra-processed foods is designed to stimulate overeating, because these foods are cheap, profitable, and convenient. When companies sell more ultra-processed foods, they make more money. The unfortunate side effect (for you) is that they also cause weight gain. Eating these foods also makes us feel better because they stimulate the reward centers of our brain. Because of the comfort we get when eating them, some people use food to self-medicate their low mood. While this strategy works temporarily, it may cause long-term weight gain.

The environmental and social determinants of eating behavior are likely the most important topics related to weight gain that are never discussed. Our eating behavior is inextricably shaped by our surroundings, family, and friends. When people move from an area with low obesity to one with high obesity, they gain weight. Why? Because they begin to reflect the eating habits and attitudes of their environment. These social and cultural norms are transmitted through social modeling and peer groups that influence our mindset and our eating habits.

To effectively deal with the three types of hunger, we need to follow the time-tested and ancient Golden Rules of weight loss. To put them into practice, follow the weight-loss tips throughout the book. For a recap of these tips, see page 231.

PART ONE

Homeostatic Hunger

1

DEBUNKING THE
CALORIE DELUSION

"IT IS TIME to share a striking, and not widely appreciated, secret," wrote Dr. Dariush Mozaffarian, dean emeritus at the Tufts University School of Medicine and director of the Tufts Food Is Medicine Institute, in 2022. Trained at Stanford, Columbia, and Harvard, he has taught at Harvard and Tufts University, served on the President's Council on Sports, Fitness, and Nutrition, and is one of the most cited nutrition researchers in the world. So it's worth paying attention to what he says.

What is this "striking" secret? **The reason we gain weight is far more complex than just eating too many calories.** Writing about obesity, Dr. Mozaffarian said: "The commonly accepted explanation is pervasive overeating: ever-increasing energy intake as the population gains weight, year after year. However, evidence does not support this hypothesis."[1]

Take note: science says that weight gain is not simply the result of eating "too much." Therefore, just eating less will likely not lead to successful weight loss. We've all pretended this Eat Less strategy works but, deep down, we know it doesn't. Every scientific study has proved it. Millions of people have tried, yet the rate of obesity in the U.S. has skyrocketed even as Americans ate fewer calories and exercised more (Eat Less, Move More). The same outcome holds true in countries all around the world.

SEPARATING SCIENCE FROM SUGGESTION

NO WONDER WE'RE CONFUSED. Our eyes, our bodies, science, common sense, and logic tell us that counting and cutting calories doesn't work for weight loss. Our governments, our health organizations, and our TVs tell us that it does. For example, in 2024, the U.S. Department of Agriculture stated on its website at Nutrition.gov: "Weight loss can be achieved either by eating fewer calories or by burning more calories with physical activity, preferably both" (Figure 1.1).[2] The American Heart Association's scientific statement from 2021 asserts that to lose weight, you must "adjust energy intake and expenditure."[3] The *Handbook of Obesity*, a two-volume reference guide written by global experts that covers the basic science of obesity, could not be clearer: "A decrease in energy intake is the most important dietary component of weight loss and maintenance." It confidently proclaims that "a decrease of 500–1000 kcal/d will produce a weight loss of 1–2 lbs/week."[4]

Figure 1.1. Statement on the U.S. Department of Agriculture's Nutrition.gov website about weight loss

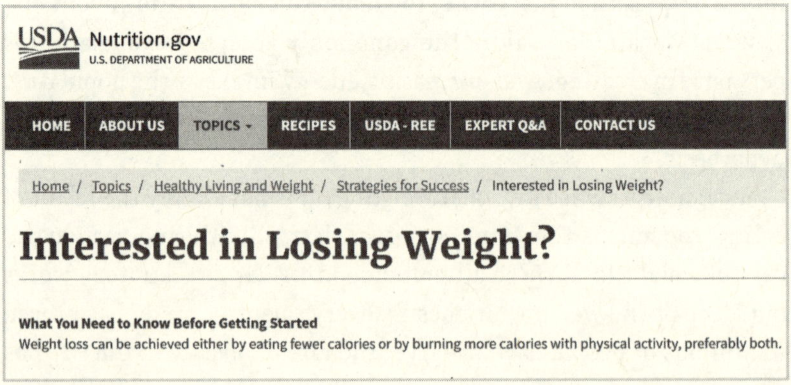

USDA Nutrition.gov
U.S. DEPARTMENT OF AGRICULTURE

HOME | ABOUT US | TOPICS ▾ | RECIPES | USDA - REE | EXPERT Q&A | CONTACT US

Home / Topics / Healthy Living and Weight / Strategies for Success / Interested in Losing Weight?

Interested in Losing Weight?

What You Need to Know Before Getting Started
Weight loss can be achieved either by eating fewer calories or by burning more calories with physical activity, preferably both.

But this advice doesn't work. It never has, and it never will. Dr. Jeffrey Flier, former dean of the Faculty of Medicine at Harvard University, and Dr. Eleftheria Maratos-Flier, an endocrinologist and emerita professor of medicine at the same school, wrote: "Successful treatment of obesity... is rarely achievable in clinical practice," and "long-term success is infrequent regardless of the approach."[5] Jeez Louise. This treatment to eat fewer calories and burn more of them almost never works! Dr. Flier and Dr. Maratos-Flier said so, and we all know this is the truth. Why is "eating fewer calories" a cornerstone of therapy if we also know that this treatment almost always fails?

Just how bad is this standard weight-loss advice? If you are overweight or obese, only one in thirty-seven people, or 2.7 percent, achieve a normal body mass index (BMI), a standard measurement of obesity.[6] That's a 97.3 percent failure rate.

And the news gets worse. If you are one of the estimated 42 percent of Americans who is classified as obese (body mass index over 30), then your rate of success plummets to 0.65 percent. The failure rate is **99.35 percent**! Shut the front door.

And the news gets worse still, because of relapses. Even if you get to a normal body mass index, it does little good if you don't stay there. A whopping 43 percent of people don't maintain that healthy weight over three years, which means the true success rate for "eating fewer calories" is about 0.37 percent. That's a **99.63 percent** failure rate. Oh. My. Goodness.

But you already knew this strategy didn't work. You've tried it. I've tried it. Friends and family have tried it. It hasn't worked for anybody. As I showed in *The Obesity Code*, every scientific study proved it didn't work.

The Women's Health Initiative observational study, one of the largest randomized controlled trials ever done, reduced participants' caloric intake by 371 calories per day and increased their physical activity by 10 percent. Eat Less, Move More, right? Did these women thank their "experts" as the pounds flew off their bodies as promised? Hardly. After seven years of dieting, they did not weigh any less than the women in the study who didn't change their diet at all. Calorie counters should have expected over 30 pounds (13.6 kg) of weight loss per year!

What about health benefits beyond weight loss, like reducing heart disease and stroke? Oh dear, there's more bad news. The study targeting weight loss "achieved primarily through reduction of caloric intake" funded by the National Institutes of Health and conducted by the Look AHEAD Research Group was one of the longest and the largest studies ever done in nutrition science.[7] Did it work? Hell to the no. In October 2012, the trial was stopped early for the reason of... futility.[8] Eight long years of calorie restriction (1200 cal/day) did not reduce heart disease or stroke, or improve diabetes, so the trial was stopped. And the cost of this futile treatment? An estimated $2864.60 per person in the first year, and $1119.80 each year after that.[9] Because this expensive and massive study does not support the "cut your calories" narrative, it is almost never discussed.

In 2022, the multimillion-dollar Reach Ahead for Lifestyle and Health (REAL HEALTH) diabetes study showed once again that calorie-restricted diets did not produce lasting weight loss.[10] Ouch.

Cutting calories *sounds* like it should help you should lose weight and be healthier, but it does not. Science only proves what everybody already knew. I'm just saying the quiet part out loud. The emperor has no clothes. Calorie-restriction diets for weight loss have a perfect track record, unblemished by success. Why? There are two possible answers:

1. The advice is good, but the people are bad. They can't or won't follow the advice.
2. The advice is bad.

"Experts" blame the victim, which leads to fat shaming. However, the inconvenient truth stares us in the face. If you are one of the 99.63 percent of people who have tried calorie restriction and failed to lose weight, remember this: you were expected to fail. The doctors, the scientists, the dieticians, the "experts" all *knew* you would fail. The advice was bad.

Here's the thing. It doesn't matter if scientists *think* that calorie restriction should work. Test it, and if it doesn't work, then accept that it doesn't work. Move forward. That's the way of science.

DIGGING DEEPER THAN A SINGLE FACTOR

DR. MOZAFFARIAN ALLUDED to the problem: obesity results from many important factors other than simply the number of calories. In the 1970s, there was little obesity despite plenty of food being available. You know what people *didn't* do? Count calories. In the 2020s, obesity is a worldwide epidemic. You know what people obsess about? Counting calories.

The idea that weight gain is all about calories appeals to our desire for a simple explanation. Think of this idea like a common currency. If everyone uses the U.S. dollar as a measure of currency and exchange, then items as different as a plane ticket or an onion can be measured in the same units. The plane ticket is expensive and costs more dollars. The onion is cheaper and costs fewer dollars. We often think that calories are the common currency of foods: brownies contain many calories and broccoli has fewer calories. We imagine, therefore, that these different foods can be measured on the same currency of calories. The more calories you eat, the more body fat you will gain. That's the story we've all been told. It's wildly incorrect.

Calories are a measure of heat energy contained in food. That's a useful concept in physics, but not in physiology. It provides no information about the body's all-important hormonal response to those foods and is therefore a sadly incomplete description of the fattening effect of that food.

Most human diseases are multifactorial. Bacteria may cause an infection, but other factors, such as underlying immune status, hygiene, and stress, are important too. Age may play a role in heart disease, but gender, hypertension, diabetes, physical activity, and family history are all important factors too. Why would obesity be any different? Why is obesity *only* about calories? Identifying and understanding the other factors that lead to weight gain and obesity can only make weight-loss treatment more successful. We might include, for example, processing of foods, timing of meals, frequency of meals, macronutrient content of meals, fiber intake, speed of absorption, emotional eating, food addiction, societal influences, social norms, and eating habits.

As we will see, the number of calories you eat is a single factor in weight gain, but not the only one—and I would argue, not the most important one. If we look at the eight countries in the world that eat the most calories and simply compare the number of calories eaten to the obesity rate, you'll quickly notice some odd facts (Table 1.1[11]). People in Bahrain eat more calories each day than people in the U.S., but they have less obesity. The Irish eat a mere 17 fewer calories per day than the Americans, but Ireland has almost 30 percent less obesity. The Austrians eat more calories daily than the Germans, but they have almost a third less obesity. The Belgians eat more calories than the Turks but have less obesity.[12]

Table 1.1. Number of calories eaten per day versus obesity globally, 2022

Country	Calories per day	Obesity rate
Bahrain	4012	37.2%
USA	3868	42.9%
Ireland	3851	30.8%
Belgium	3824	22%
Turkey	3762	34.2%
Austria	3739	17%
Germany	3648	24.2%
Italy	3621	21.6%
Correlation coefficient 0.6		

8

The correlation coefficient shows us the strength of the relationship between the two variables (calories eaten and obesity rate). While the correlation is positive, meaning that the two variables do affect each other, it is not particularly strong. When calculated for 156 countries, the correlation is 0.6, which suggests that 40 percent or so of the obesity rate is explained by something other than total number of calories eaten.

Calories are a measure of energy. Food provides our bodies with energy (calories), but it also contains *information*. Our body responds to the foods we eat by releasing hormones. Equal calorie portions of two different foods (like cookies versus eggs) generate two completely different hormonal responses. Hormones are the chemical messengers that tell our bodies how to react, so our bodies react very differently, even though the calories are the same.

For example, 200 calories of cookies spike the blood glucose and the hormone insulin, whereas 200 calories of eggs do not. Why pretend this difference does not matter? It's as bizarre as saying that money is money, so selling cocaine and selling men's suits is the same thing. In reality, there are so many other consequential differences.

Food contains two important things:

1. Energy (calories)
2. Information

Different foods provoke different hormones that provide the body with instructions as to what to do with that energy. Those instructions could be to burn those calories or to store them as body fat. To lose weight, we must also focus on the hormones.

UNDERSTANDING THE ENERGY BALANCE EQUATION

9

ENERGY STORED EQUALS **Energy In** minus **Energy Out**. For our body, food energy is stored as body fat and measured in calories. So the Energy Balance Equation looks like this:

Body Fat = Calories In – Calories Out

This equation is always true, but it doesn't mean what most of us think it does. Let's rewrite the equation this way:

Calories In = Body Fat + Calories Out

Writing it this way shows that for every calorie you eat, your body may either

1. store it (as body fat) or
2. burn it (for energy).

Whether or not you store body fat depends more on what your body *does* with the calories, rather than simply the total number of calories. If you *eat* fewer calories, your body does not necessarily *store* fewer calories (less body fat). It may instead *burn* fewer calories, and this does not contradict the Energy Balance Equation. Eating calories and storing calories are two fundamentally different issues.

Which path does your body choose? Store it or burn it? This is the most, most important question. It's the hormones that decide. If insulin is high, then the calorie is stored. If insulin is low, then it is burned for energy. Therefore, the most important aspect of weight loss is the hormones.

Think about money. You earn it (Money In), spend it (Money Out), and save some (Money Saved, such as in the bank). If you've earned a lot of money, it doesn't necessarily mean that you've saved a lot. You can earn a lot and save only a little. You can also earn a little and save a lot. These scenarios are related but not necessarily the same thing. The same is true with calories. If you eat fewer calories, you won't necessarily store less body fat.

Again, body fat is merely a store of food energy (calories). What controls the storage or release of calories? It's not the total number of calories. It's the hormones. Here's the simple science of weight loss:

1. Body fat is a way that the body stores food energy (calories).
2. Hormones, especially insulin, tell the body fat whether it should store or release calories.
3. Foods provoke hormonal responses that tell our body whether to store or release calories from storage (body fat).
4. Losing weight depends on changing the hormones so that body fat is released instead of being stored.

Let me illustrate the Energy Balance Equation with a parable.

The parable of the warehouse manager (and how it relates to weight loss)

Suppose you own a store that sells, say... lumber. Every day, you buy about 2000 pounds of lumber and sell about 2000 pounds.

You have a warehouse to store lumber. If you sell a bit more lumber one day, you take some from the warehouse. If you sell a bit less lumber, you store the extra in the warehouse. (In your body, you eat about 2000 calories and burn about 2000 calories. Body fat is a warehouse for calories, in case you have a surplus or deficit.) All good.

The warehouse manager receives every daily shipment along with instructions about how much lumber to store or release. (In your body, insulin is the warehouse manager and controls the "warehouse" of body fat. When you eat, insulin goes up and you store calories. When you don't eat, insulin goes down and you release calories. Different foods release different amounts of insulin.) All good.

One day, you notice the warehouse is overflowing with lumber. There is so much extra wood that it is stored outside where it is rotting. You estimate there are 175,000 extra pounds of lumber in storage. That's not good. (In your body, you carry an extra 50 pounds of body fat, which is about 175,000 of excess stored calories and is becoming a big health problem.)

The warehouse manager has been getting instructions to store more lumber than usual, which has thrown off the normal balance.

11

Either the daily deliveries are larger than usual or the deliveries are the same size but more lumber from each delivery is being stored. Both are possible. (Insulin levels are higher than normal, which tells the body to store more calories. Either you are eating more calories or you're eating the same number of calories but storing more than usual. Both are possible.)

So, you hire a consultant, who shows you a fancy presentation. They say: "Well, it's very simple. Too much stored lumber is simply a lumber balance problem, which is governed by the lumber balance equation:

Lumber Stored = Lumber In – Lumber Out

"The First Law of Thermodynamics for Lumber says that lumber cannot be created or destroyed. To reduce stored lumber, buy less lumber or sell more lumber. Simple. Lumber In, Lumber Out. That'll be $12 million, please."

But the solution is fundamentally flawed because it forgets that, ultimately, the warehouse manager controls how much lumber is stored or released. (In your body, people say it's all about the Energy Balance Equation, Body Fat = Calories In – Calories Out, but they forget that the calories stored (body fat) is controlled by hormones like insulin.)

Relieved to have a logical-sounding solution, you immediately buy less lumber: 1500 pounds instead of the usual 2000 pounds. You hope you'll still sell 2000 pounds, and that the extra 500 pounds will be released from the warehouse. But the warehouse manager's instructions haven't changed, so they don't release extra lumber. With only 1500 pounds of lumber coming in, you can only sell 1500 pounds. Not good. (In your body, you eat 500 fewer calories per day, but insulin hasn't changed, so body fat is not released, and you compensate by burning 500 fewer calories. Eat less, burn less. Not good.)

Certain that this Lumber In, Lumber Out solution is total crap, you hire a new consultant. They say the same: it's all about Lumber In,

12

Lumber Out. Just buy less and sell more. The instructions to the warehouse manager are irrelevant. (In your body, everybody insists that weight loss is all about Calories In, Calories Out, completely disregarding the well-known hormonal impact of foods.)

You try the Lumber In, Lumber Out strategy again and again, but it fails every single time. All your colleagues have tried the same strategy but also failed. Your consultant says: "It must work. It's a scientific certainty, so the problem must be with you. You are a liar. You don't want to solve the problem badly enough. You don't have the willpower. You disgust me." (In your body, you try cutting calories again and again, only to fail every single time. Everybody around you silently condemns your lack of willpower or some other character defect. You believe it's all your fault and that you are the problem.)

The manager still controls the warehouse and is still getting instructions to store more lumber. The most important factor in adjusting the inventory is the warehouse manager's instructions. Lumber In and Lumber Out only indirectly influence warehouse storage. (In your body, hormones directly control the storage or release of food energy (calories) into body fat. Therefore, hormones are the most important factor in weight loss. Calories In and Calories Out only indirectly affect Body Fat. As Bill Clinton might have quipped: "It's the Insulin, stupid.")

RECOGNIZING THE ROLE OF HORMONES IN WEIGHT LOSS

HORMONES ARE THE most important factor in determining body weight. This fact shouldn't come as a surprise, since virtually all aspects of our body are run by hormones. For example:

- Hormones tell us to be hungry (for example, ghrelin)
- Hormones tell us to be full (for example, GLP-1, GIP, peptide YY, cholecystokinin)
- Hormones tell us to use more energy (for example, norepinephrine)
- Hormones tell us to grow (for example, human growth hormone)

13

- Hormones tell us to lose body fat (for example, leptin)
- Hormones tell us to gain more body fat (for example, insulin, cortisol)

Don't worry, we'll discuss all these hormones later in the book (see Chapter 4).

When you eat, insulin levels rise. Insulin tells the body to store calories (body fat) and not to release calories. Insulin inhibits lipolysis, which is a fancy way to say that high insulin levels block fat burning.

When you don't eat (fasting), insulin levels fall. Fasting lowers insulin, which tells your body to release calories from storage (body fat). **You can't release calories from body fat storage unless the insulin "brake" is released.**

How much you eat (the number of calories) and the hormonal response are related, but they are not the same thing. Some foods stimulate more insulin than others. In other words, **some foods are more fattening than others** (Figure 1.2[13]). That statement doesn't seem outrageous to me. Cookies are more fattening than broccoli. Candy is more fattening than eggs. Seems right, yet the nutritional orthodoxy reacts like I've just urinated on the White House lawn. They insist that if two foods have equal calories, they are equally fattening. But nutritional orthodoxy completely ignores the hormonal aspect of the food eaten.

Figure 1.2. All these foods contain 200 calories, but they are not equally fattening

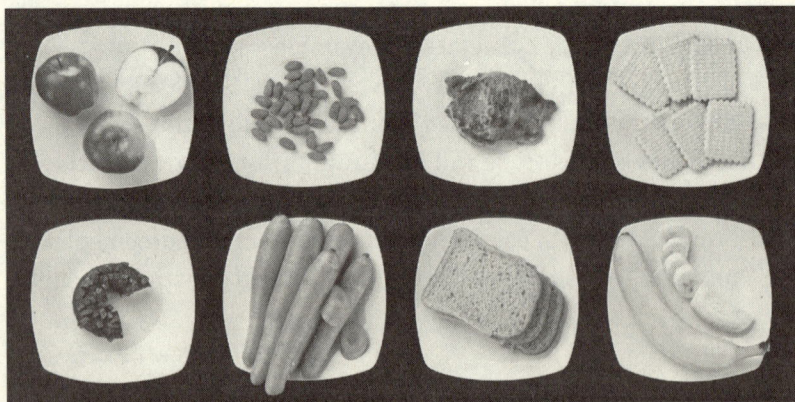

Is it really both calories *and* hormones? Not really. It's *all* hormones. Think about the three variables we care about, as outlined in the Energy Balance Equation:

1. Calories In
2. Calories Out
3. Calories Stored (Body Fat)

What determines how many calories we eat (Calories In)? We like to pretend this number is purely our choice, but this belief is false. We eat more if we are hungry and less if we are full. Hunger is determined by our hormones, among other things.

What determines how many calories are burned (Calories Out)? Metabolic rate, with a small amount used for exercise. We don't decide our metabolic rate, our hormones do.

What determines how much body fat is stored (Calories Stored)? Again, it is our hormones, mostly insulin.

How much we eat, how much we burn, and how much gets stored in body fat are all driven by our hormones. So why pretend that the different hormonal response to different foods makes no difference and only the number of calories does? For weight loss, there are good calories and there are bad calories because of the associated hormonal "instructions."

Consider a hypothetical situation. Suppose you eat 2000 calories per day (Calories In) and burn 2000 calories per day (Calories Out). Your body fat (Calories Stored) remains stable (Figure 1.3).

Figure 1.3. When Calories In equals Calories Out, body fat is stable

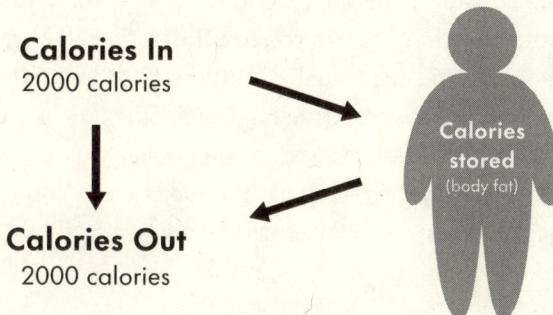

Calories In
2000 calories

Calories Out
2000 calories

Calories stored (body fat)

15

Now you want to lose body fat, so you eat fewer calories, say 1500 calories per day. But you eat highly refined carbohydrates and very frequently. Insulin stays high, which prevents the release of calories from body fat stores. Insulin inhibits lipolysis (insulin blocks fat burning). Only 1500 calories are available to burn, so your body must burn fewer calories, 1500. You generate less body heat, so you feel cold. Your brain gets less energy, so you feel sluggish. Your basal metabolic rate is slowing, and you feel lethargic. Worse, you are not losing body fat. In this case, when insulin remains high, you eat fewer calories *and* you burn fewer calories, but calories stored (body fat) stays the same (Figure 1.4).

Figure 1.4. When Calories In equals Calories Out but insulin is high, body fat increases

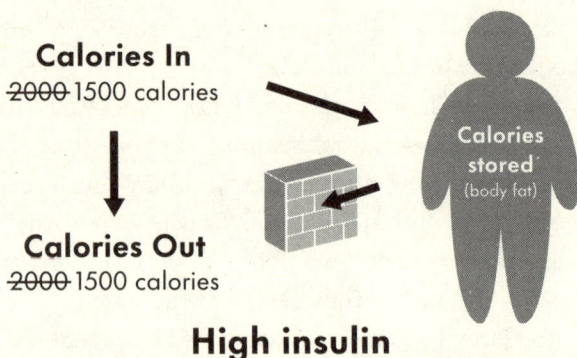

Calories In
~~2000~~ 1500 calories

Calories Out
~~2000~~ 1500 calories

Calories stored (body fat)

High insulin

You aren't losing weight, so everybody thinks you must be cheating and eating the same number of calories (or more). They silently condemn you for your lack of willpower. "You didn't want to lose the weight badly enough," they think. You are eating fewer calories but burning fewer calories because insulin doesn't allow calories to be released from body fat. The less you eat, the less you'll burn. That's the cruel hoax of a calorie-reduced diet. Eat less, burn less. Every scientific study of weight loss has confirmed it. Not good.

Now consider an alternative situation for weight loss. You eat fewer calories (1500 per day) by eating natural foods and incorporating regular fasting intervals. Insulin levels drop. Now, when insulin is low, your

16

body can release 500 calories from storage (body fat) to make up for the 500 fewer calories you are eating. You still burn 2000 calories (Figure 1.5).

Figure 1.5. When Calories In equals Calories Out but insulin is low, body fat decreases

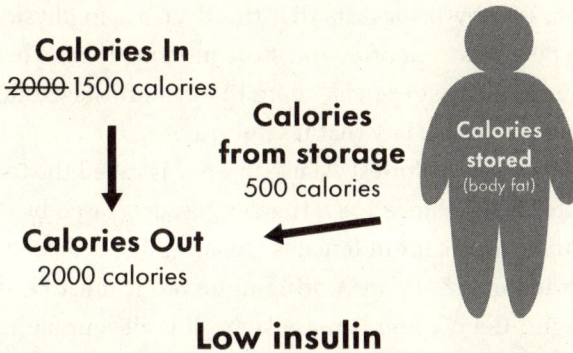

Calories In
~~2000~~ 1500 calories

Calories from storage
500 calories

Calories stored (body fat)

Calories Out
2000 calories

Low insulin

In both situations, you have eaten 1500 calories. In the first situation, you didn't lose body fat and in the second situation you did. What was the difference? The hormones. Whether insulin is high or low makes *all* the difference.

If you focus only on the calories and ignore the hormones, you'll never solve the fat storage problem. Remember, food contains two things: the energy (calories) *and* the instructions for what to do with those calories. You must understand both.

The calorie delusion is that obesity is purely a caloric imbalance. The truth is that obesity is not merely a caloric imbalance but a hormonal one.

Tip #1: Don't count calories.

Tip #2: Understand that foods contain both calories and information about what to do with those calories.

REJECTING THE EXERCISE MYTH

A COMMON MYTH suggests that obesity is caused by the many conveniences of modern living. We used to walk, but now we take the car instead. We used to take the stairs, but now we use the elevator. The list goes on. The myth suggests that this decrease in physical activity means we burn fewer calories and store more body fat. Therefore, we believe, we should just exercise more to burn off those calories. This myth sounds plausible. Pity that it's not true.

The total energy (calories) we use in a day is called the total energy expenditure, or TEE. Since 1982, the TEE has decreased by 7.7 percent in males and 5.6 percent in females globally. Aha! People are burning fewer calories and therefore storing more fat. It must be the lack of exercise, right? Get off your lazy ass, right? It is all your fault, right?

Wrong.

Calories spent exercising has *increased* steadily over the past forty years. The decline in TEE was driven by an even greater **decrease in metabolic rate**. Metabolic rate is the speed at which your body uses energy, or the rate at which your body burns calories. We cannot control this rate. You can't decide how much heat your body generates. You can't decide how much energy your brain, heart, kidneys, or lungs use. A decrease in metabolic rate is not due to lack of willpower or self-control. The rate—up or down—is controlled by, you guessed it, hormones. So, yes, people are burning fewer calories; but, no, that decrease isn't due to lack of exercise.[14]

For a moderately active person, metabolic rate is by far the most important component of TEE. A rough breakdown:

- 70% resting metabolic rate
- 20% physical activity
- 10% diet-induced thermogenesis[15]

Our resting metabolic rate (RMR) is the amount of energy the body needs to function while at rest. RMR includes the energy we need to breathe, keep our kidneys and brain working, maintain our body temperature, and so on. Physical activity includes any movement that's part of our daily activities, including walking, cooking, and taking the stairs, as well as dedicated exercise, such as going for a run or doing a yoga class or spending time at the gym. And diet-induced thermogenesis is a fancy way of describing the energy we need to digest our food.

So can't you simply crank up the physical activity (exercise) to lose weight? Uh, no. When you exercise more, your body compensates by reducing the calories it spends on metabolic rate (Figure 1.6). Exercising more than a moderate amount, about thirty minutes per day or so, does not increase total calories expended. Why? Because your body becomes more energy efficient the more you exercise it. Heart rate slows down. You feel more relaxed. Blood pressure drops. Those are all good things, but the body uses *less* energy and therefore burns fewer calories.[16]

Figure 1.6. As physical activity increases, metabolic rate decreases and total energy expenditure stays the same

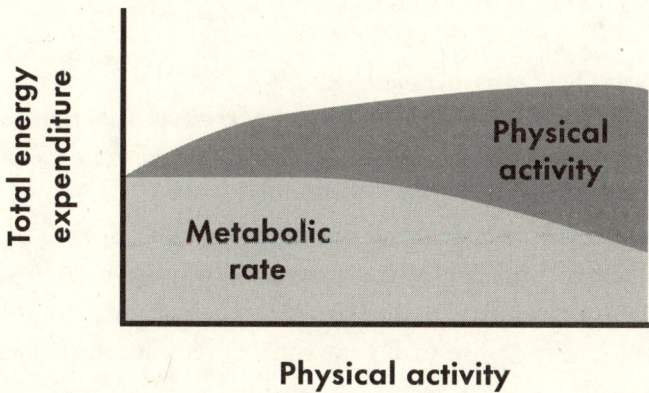

High levels of exercise also increase hunger, which means your body wants more calories. They don't call it "working up an appetite" for no reason, you know.[17] I won't belabor this point, since physical activity is clearly highly beneficial for health and most people should be doing

more. However, exercise shouldn't be the focus of your weight-loss plan. Remember, obesity is a multifactorial disease.

> **Tip #3:** Exercise for its many health benefits,
> but not for weight loss.

ANSWERING THE "THREE WHYS" OF WEIGHT GAIN

THERE IS A CONCEPT in logic known as the "three whys": to understand the root of a problem, ask the question "Why?" at least three times. For example, a child might ask, "Why do I need to go to school?" The usual answer is "So you can learn stuff," which typically elicits a response like, "When will I ever need to know the capital of Uganda?" or "When will I ever need to calculate the area of a circle?" I suppose these questions aren't unreasonable, because our answer hasn't satisfied the child's root desire to know why. Instead, we should invite more follow-up questions. For example, answering the "three whys" in this case might elicit the following exchange:

1. *Why do I need to go to school?* Because you will learn things.
2. *Why do I need to learn things?* Because you can get a better job.
3. *Why do I need a better job?* Because you can make more money.

Aha! A child can understand the simple logic of "Go to school now to make more money later." After asking three "whys," you get close to the root of the problem. If you stop thinking at the superficial, most obvious, answer to the first or second "why," you'll never solve the problem.

Consider the *Titanic*. Why did that ship sink? The usual, most obvious, answer is, "Because it hit an iceberg." This answer is technically correct, but it's not useful because it fails to identify the root cause. This shallow understanding can only lead to useless advice not to hit icebergs during future voyages.

Instead, ask the "three whys":

1. *Why did the* Titanic *sink?* Because it hit an iceberg.
2. *Why did it hit an iceberg?* Because the captain didn't see it in time to avoid it.
3. *Why didn't they see it?* Because the *Titanic* was going too fast.

Aha! This series of questions allows us to clarify the root cause: If the captain had slowed down, they might have seen the iceberg and been able to avoid it. A useful lesson we can draw from that is "Slow down in bad weather" rather than "Don't hit icebergs." This more useful advice comes from thinking more deeply and applying the "three whys."

Calorie counting is shallow thinking that stops at the first why. That's the reason it doesn't work.

For weight loss, the first "why" we ask is:

1. *Why do we gain weight?* Because we eat more calories than we burn. If you stop thinking here, at the level of the first "why," you get the solution "Eat fewer calories than you burn." That's the simplistic and useless "Don't hit icebergs" solution or the "To learn stuff" answer. This first-order thinking is simply not useful, as proven by decades of futile weight-loss advice.

   It's true that when Calories In > Calories Out, you gain body fat. But I'm not interested *that* Calories In > Calories Out. I know that already. I'm interested to know *why* Calories In > Calories Out. Nobody is *trying* to eat more calories. That leads to the second "why."

   For weight loss, the second "why" we ask is:

2. *Why do we eat more calories than we burn?* Because we're **hungry**. Now we are getting closer to the root cause: hunger, not calories. Trying to lose weight by reducing calories without addressing the root cause of the hunger is doomed to fail. The main problem when you simply eat less is that hunger increases. Those two goals are diametrically opposed: you are trying to eat less, but your hunger

is trying to make you eat more. Something will eventually have to give. Usually, your unruly hunger wins and you eat more despite your best intentions. Which leads us to our third "why."

For weight loss, the third "why" we ask is:

3. *Why are we hungry?* This question is critical, and yet the answer has almost nothing to do with calories. The root cause of "overeating" might better be explored as the problem of "over-hunger." Why are we hungry? This answer is not so simple, because there are *three* fundamentally distinct types of hunger that drive our eating behavior. Each type of hunger has different causes and treatments.

Remember the three types of hunger, all of which may cause weight gain (Figure 1.7):

1. Homeostatic hunger
2. Hedonic hunger
3. Conditioned hunger

Figure 1.7. The root causes may be different, but all types of hunger can lead to weight gain

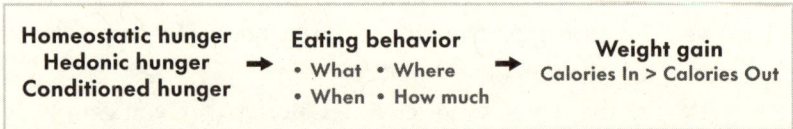

Homeostatic hunger Hedonic hunger Conditioned hunger	➡	Eating behavior • What • Where • When • How much	➡	Weight gain Calories In > Calories Out

Homeostatic hunger maintains adequate nutrition and avoids excessive weight gain. Homeostasis is a self-regulating system to maintain a stable weight; that is, our body has a fat thermostat. Hormones adjust that thermostat up or down. Homeostatic hunger is regulated largely by hormones.

Hedonic hunger is driven by pleasure-seeking behavior. Eating is rewarding, pleasurable, and makes us feel good, no matter what our body fat percentage or the nutritional quality of the food.

Conditioned hunger includes the food environment and social aspects of eating behavior. Conditioned hunger is both shaped by the environment around us and caused by the habits we learn and accrue over our lifetime.

Consider how each type of hunger would answer the question "Why are you eating?"

- Homeostatic hunger would say: "Because I'm hungry." *Cue stomach growling*. Homeostatic hunger is the hunger you satisfy when your stomach growls or your energy level drops.
- Hedonic hunger would say: "Because food makes me feel better" or "Because it looks so good." Hedonic hunger is the hunger you satisfy with dessert. You are not hungry in a physical sense, but you want to eat dessert for the pure pleasure of it.
- Conditioned hunger would say: "Because it is lunchtime." This is the baloney sandwich you eat at lunch, not because you are hungry or because it looks delicious, but simply because it is lunchtime and you are in the habit of eating lunch.

Hunger and satiety are not choices. You can choose what and how much you eat, but you can't choose to be less hungry. You cannot choose to see that tempting dessert as less tempting. The advice to eat less is useless without advice on how to reduce hunger. It's as ridiculous as saying to somebody "Don't worry" and expecting them to not worry.

Knowing why we gain weight can help us to devise effective solutions to lose it and keep it off. Knowing the root causes can also help us to prevent weight gain in the first place. To do that, we need to know more about each of the root causes.

| 2 |

REGULATING THE
BODY FAT THERMOSTAT

I N 1968, Dr. Ethan Sims conducted a series of studies with people incarcerated at the Vermont State Prison. For half a year, the research team fed them up to 10,000 calories a day, with the goal of experimentally inducing obesity. During the overfeeding phase, the average weight gain per person was 35 pounds (16 kg), mostly due to an increase in fat. However, just ten weeks after the study finished, everyone had returned to their baseline weight.

While unethical by today's standards, Dr. Sims's overfeeding experiment with incarcerated people revealed that simply increasing calorie intake generally does not cause long-term weight gain. That is, the body weight of lean people, pushed to extreme overfeeding (8000 to 10,000 calories per day), did grudgingly increase but effortlessly boomeranged back to normal after the experiment finished. Dr. Sims had rediscovered the puzzling phenomenon that German scientist Rudolf Neumann termed Luxuskonsumption in 1902. Why did lean people have no problem losing weight and overweight people have so much trouble?

Legendary obesity researcher Dr. George Bray was stunned by these overfeeding studies that challenged the naïve but widely accepted notion that weight gain can be reduced to "eating too many calories."[1]

In the grand tradition of scientific self-experimentation, Bray tried to make himself gain weight. For lunch, he ate two sandwiches instead of one but found that the volume of food was "more than his stomach would allow."

Next, Dr. Bray ate more "fattening" foods to try to make himself gain weight. He selected foods high in sugar and fat, such as ice cream and milkshakes, and sure enough he found success. In ten weeks on this diet, he gained 10 kg (22 pounds). But soon he began to feel uncomfortably hot all the time. His body was generating more heat by burning more food energy (calories) to counteract his weight gain.

When Dr. Bray finished his experiment and returned to his regular diet, he quickly dropped back to his original weight. In six weeks, he lost 22 pounds and maintained that weight loss—with **no effort**! How did that happen? The answer centers on the control of the body's calorie "warehouse" and its manager (hormones). This is the effect of the body set weight or what I call the body fat thermostat.

THE CORE PRINCIPLE OF HOMEOSTASIS

THE HUMAN BODY needs a continuous supply of energy to power the brain, heart, lungs, and other organs. But food, which supplies that energy (calories), is only available episodically. To bridge the gap, the body requires a system of energy (calorie) storage, which is body fat. But how much body fat should we store? Ten thousand calories? A hundred thousand? A million? Ten million?

A popular argument suggests that humans are designed to store all available calories as body fat, and the more, the better. Now that food is easily available, goes that argument, we inevitably gain weight. It's the nature of modern life, so we must fight against our body constantly to eat fewer calories. That argument sounds logical, if you don't think about it too hard. But like a rotting watermelon, once you get past the surface layer, it stinks. Biology just doesn't work like that.

For any species to survive, body fat percentage must stay within a tight range, even though the number of calories eaten varies wildly.

25

If animals get too fat, they cannot catch food or avoid predators. If animals are too skinny, they can't survive a period of famine, such as winter. That's why adult wild animals, whether lions, tigers, elephants, fish, or any other species, are almost never obese.

The story of Joseph in the Bible recounts seven years of plenty but no ancient epidemic of morbid obesity. Lots of calories were available, but people did not mindlessly gain fat. Humanity has survived about 2 million years without having witnessed a global obesity epidemic.

If stored calories (body fat) simply reflect how many calories we eat, then it should fluctuate enormously. Our daily calorie intake varies wildly, but our body weight does not. Sometimes we eat a lot. Sometimes we eat very little. Despite this wide variance, body fat stays remarkably stable.

This stability, also seen in wild animals, cannot simply be due to managing our calorie intake. Wild deer, sharks, and wolves don't count their calories. They don't measure their metabolic rate in a lab. Yet they effortlessly maintain proper levels of body fat. Prior to 1977, humans generally maintained proper levels of body fat as well.

Today, the average American eats about 3868 calories per day and gains about 1 pound (or roughly 3500 calories) per year.[2] To only gain a pound of fat per year, a person must match their calorie intake with expenditure to an accuracy of 99.73 percent. Yet 8 billion people worldwide do this seemingly impossible task without accurately knowing how many calories they eat and how many calories they burn.

Obviously, body fat can only be maintained with such remarkable stability with an automatic control mechanism. How much body fat we carry is set at an optimal point called the body set weight. If weight rises above this point, we activate mechanisms to lose weight. If weight drops below this point, we activate mechanisms to gain weight. This automatic mechanism to maintain an internal stable environment despite external changes is called homeostasis.

Homeostasis is our body's tendency toward a balance point, or equilibrium. It is not unique to body fat percentage but applies to virtually every essential physiological process. For example, normal

26

body temperature is maintained at roughly 98 degrees Fahrenheit (37 degrees Celsius). If we live in the Sahara Desert, where it is very hot, we sweat to cool the body back to normal temperature. If we live in the North Pole, where it is very cold, we shiver, heating the body back to that same normal temperature. Either way, despite highly variable external conditions, homeostasis ensures that our body temperature is maintained in a stable range.

Homeostasis is a core biological principle. All mission-critical systems in the body are maintained automatically and involuntarily, without requiring any conscious thought. For example:

- **Hydration.** When we drink more, we pee more. When we drink less, we pee less.
- **Blood electrolyte levels.** If we eat too much sodium, potassium, or chloride, we pee it out. When we eat too few of any of these blood electrolytes, we don't pee it out.
- **Blood pH (acidity).** If our blood becomes too acidic, our kidneys dump acid (as ammonia) in the urine. If our blood is too alkaline, the kidneys dump bicarbonate to restore balance.
- **Blood glucose.** If blood glucose goes too low, we get hungry. We eat to increase blood glucose levels. If blood glucose goes too high, we pee out glucose to restore balance.
- **Oxygen and carbon dioxide.** If our blood oxygen level drops too low or carbon dioxide goes too high, we breathe faster (hyper-ventilate) to raise oxygen and lower carbon dioxide. If carbon dioxide drops too low, we breathe slower (hypo-ventilate). Blood oxygen is normally close to 100 percent so cannot go much higher.
- **Brightness.** If the light is too bright, our pupils constrict to reduce the amount entering our eyes. If the light is too dim, our pupils dilate.
- **Body fat.** If we have too much body fat, our body tries to reduce it by making us less hungry. If we have too little body fat, our body tries to gain it by making us hungrier.

If any of the body's many homeostatic mechanisms fail, we die. Consider body water, for example. It is utterly ridiculous to say that hydration is simply Water In minus Water Out, and therefore to maintain balance, we must always watch how much we drink and measure how much we urinate. Our body automatically adjusts our water intake (thirst) and water output (urine) to reach an optimal set point.

Equally, it is utterly ridiculous to say that body temperature is simply Heat In minus Heat Out, and so we must always have a personal air conditioner or heater at hand. Our body automatically adjusts heat generation (shivering) or dissipation (sweating) to reach an optimal set point. We get cold and go get a sweater. We get hot and take off that sweater.

Yet when we apply this same utterly ridiculous logic to body fat, it is considered a scientific inevitability. We believe that body fat is simply Calories In minus Calories Out, which can only be controlled through willpower. In fact, our body automatically adjusts our eating (Calories In) and energy expenditure (Calories Out) to reach an optimal set point called the body set weight. When the body set weight is set high, we get hungry. We eat and gain body fat. If we decide not to eat more, then our total energy expenditure (metabolic rate) decreases so that we gain body fat. What controls the body set weight? Hormones. Our body's hormones maintain the body set weight automatically, just like a thermostat maintains room temperature. That's why I call this mechanism the body fat thermostat.

The thermostat in our houses is a homeostatic mechanism. We set the desired room temperature and if the room gets too hot, the air conditioning comes on. If it gets too cold, the heater turns on. Either way, despite widely varying outside conditions, the room stays at the right temperature without the necessity of manually controlling Heat In versus Heat Out.

28   Body fat is controlled using the same homeostatic mechanism as a thermostat. The body sets an optimal level of fat stored, and the amount we eat (Calories In) and amount we burn (Calories Out) are adjusted to get the desired result. In other words, obesity is not a

disorder of eating too many calories; it is a disorder of the body set weight being too high. Remember the parable of the warehouse manager (Chapter 1)? The problem is not too much lumber coming into the warehouse; the problem is the lumber warehouse manager's instructions to keep storing lumber.

Here's another way to think about the problem. If you walk into a room and find it unbearably hot, would you think, "Oh, there's too much Heat In or too little Heat Out?" Or would you think, "Why is the thermostat set so high?" This is a *critical* distinction. In the first case, you would locate all the sources of heat going into and leaving the room. You might open the window, thinking that you can increase Heat Out to cool the room. Ultimately, that strategy won't work because the thermostat will crank up the heat to negate the ongoing heat loss. Instead, if you wondered why the thermostat is set so high, you'd only need to find the room thermostat and turn it down. This much easier solution is 100 times more likely to succeed.

By applying the principle of homeostasis to the body, we understand that we need to adjust the body fat thermostat down to lose weight. In other words, we must adjust our hormones, not our calories, to lower our body set weight.

HOW THE BODY FAT THERMOSTAT WORKS

VIRTUALLY EVERY NUTRITION STUDY ever done supports the existence of this homeostatic mechanism for body fat. In fact, most studies cannot be interpreted *except* with the knowledge of this body fat thermostat. Since we know that hormones regulate energy storage, we know that the body fat thermostat resides in the hormonal (endocrine) system and in the brain and nerves (neural system). These neurohormonal systems are the critical regulators of body fat percentage.

Over forty years ago, scientists discovered that you could make a rat obese by simply destroying an area of the brain called the ventromedial hypothalamus (VMH), involved in regulating energy balance.

The brain damage made the rat overeat and gain weight. Notice that overeating is *not* the root cause of the obesity. The damage to the VMH caused the obesity, which caused the overeating. The body fat thermostat was adjusted upward.

Similarly, by destroying a different area of the brain called the lateral hypothalamus (LH), which regulates feeding behavior, rats become anorectic and lose weight. Once again, notice that undereating is *not* the root cause of the weight loss. Rather, the brain damage decreased the body fat thermostat, which caused the rats to undereat to lose the weight they were being ordered to lose.[3]

The body fat thermostat explains Dr. Bray's puzzle of why lean people could easily lose weight whereas previously obese people could not. The difference was in the setting of their body fat thermostat. Lean people had their body fat thermostat set to "lean." After the forced weight gain, they effortlessly returned to that lean weight. Overweight people have their thermostat set to "overweight." When they lose weight, their body compels them to regain that weight.

Yes, Dr. Bray lost the weight by eating fewer calories than he was burning. That's not the question. The question is *why* he was eating fewer calories. His body fat thermostat noted that his body weight was too high and killed his appetite for several weeks until his body weight returned to normal. Dr. Bray experienced effortless weight loss.

In 1995, Dr. Rudolph Leibel elegantly confirmed this concept of the body fat thermostat in a study measuring the effect of changes in body weight on energy expended.[4] When participants were forced to overeat to gain 10 percent body weight, their metabolic rate increased by 16 percent. Their bodies were burning an extra 500 calories per day to try to reduce weight back to baseline, just as the body fat thermostat predicts. When participants then lost 10 percent body weight, their metabolic rate decreased by 15 percent. Their bodies burned fewer calories to increase their weight back to baseline, also precisely as the body fat thermostat predicts. By contrast, the Calories In, Calories Out model predicts no change in metabolic rate.

Similarly, when people are given a drug (canagliflozin) that makes them lose 300 to 400 calories of glucose through their urine daily, they lose barely any weight. Why? They spontaneously eat 300 to 400 more calories per day, just as predicted by the body fat thermostat.[5] By contrast, the Calories In, Calories Out model would expect the loss of a pound of body fat every eight or nine days, which didn't happen.

Doesn't your body get "used" to the new weight and use that as the new set weight? No. If you set your room thermostat at 72 degrees Fahrenheit (22 degrees Celsius), but keep the door open so that the room is always at 65 degrees Fahrenheit (18 degrees Celsius), does your thermostat reset after a while? No. The room thermostat will continue trying to warm up the room as long as the temperature is too low. The only solution is to adjust the room thermostat. If your body fat thermostat is set too high, you'll always try to get to that higher weight. Using willpower, you can decide to eat fewer calories, but **you can't decide to be less hungry or increase your metabolic rate.** The only way to stop fighting your body is to adjust the thermostat.

A room that is too hot is caused by a thermostat set at too high a level. The thermostat increases the heater (increased Heat In) to achieve this high temperature (Figure 2.1). The problem can only be fixed by adjusting this setting.

Figure 2.1. When you turn the room thermostat up, the room gets hotter

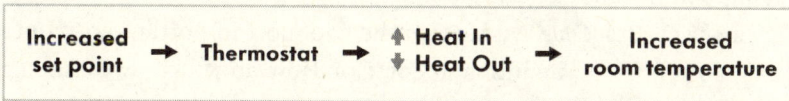

| Increased set point | → | Thermostat | → | ↑ Heat In ↓ Heat Out | → | Increased room temperature |

The root cause of obesity is the increased set point of the body fat thermostat, which increases hunger or decreases our metabolic rate to achieve the higher body weight (Figure 2.2). This problem can only be fixed by adjusting the set point back down, not by adjusting Calories In or Calories Out.

Figure 2.2. When you turn your body fat thermostat up, body fat increases

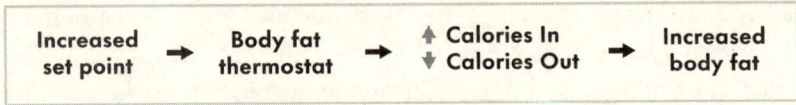

Increased set point	→	Body fat thermostat	→	↑ Calories In ↓ Calories Out	→	Increased body fat

The core questions of obesity, then, are "Why is the set point so high?" and "How do we dial it back down?" The answer to why the body fat thermostat goes up or down, like practically everything in human physiology, is hormones. Some hormones increase the body fat thermostat. Some hormones decrease the body fat thermostat.

HOW TO ADJUST THE BODY FAT THERMOSTAT

IN THE CALORIES IN, Calories Out model, we think eating fewer calories will reduce body fat. But long term, it doesn't. Why? Because it is shallow first-order thinking. You will initially lose weight and the body fat thermostat senses this change. It responds by instructing our body to regain that lost weight. How? Either hunger rises (increased Calories In) or metabolic rate falls (decreased Calories Out), or some combination of the two.[6] Virtually every scientific study of weight loss in the past century has confirmed this response. It's not some voodoo psychology; it's basic human physiology with measurable, identifiable changes in the body's hormones.

In *The Obesity Code*, we covered the two most important hormones that cause obesity: **insulin** and **cortisol**. How do we know these hormones cause obesity? Suppose we think that one thing (let's call it Factor A) causes another (let's call it Result B), how would we prove it? It's quite straightforward. We increase or decrease Factor A and observe what happens to Result B.

32

- If we give people insulin, they gain weight. If we reduce insulin (like untreated type 1 diabetes), people lose weight. Therefore, insulin is an important causal factor in weight gain/loss.

- If we give people cortisol, they gain weight. If people have too little cortisol (like adrenal insufficiency), they lose weight. Cortisol is an important causal factor for weight gain/loss.

In this book, we continue our exploration of the other neurohormonal systems that affect body fat, including

- **Leptin.** People without leptin cannot stop eating and become morbidly obese. Leptin is important for weight gain/loss.
- **Stomach distention (vagus nerve).** If we fill the stomach (with diseases like a bezoar), people lose weight. Therefore, distending the stomach and activating the vagus nerve is important for weight gain/loss.
- **Incretins (glucagon-like peptide 1 (GLP-1), glucose-dependent insulinotropic polypeptide (GIP)).** If we increase the incretin hormones (using drugs like semaglutide (Ozempic) or tirzepatide (Mounjaro)), people lose weight. Therefore, incretins are important for weight gain/loss.
- **Sympathetic tone (adrenaline, noradrenaline).** If we stimulate the sympathetic nervous system (with drugs like nicotine, amphetamines, or fenfluramine), people lose weight. If we block the sympathetic nervous system (with drugs like beta blockers), people gain weight. Therefore, sympathetic tone—the level of activity in the sympathetic nervous system—is important for weight gain/loss.
- **Sex hormones (testosterone, estrogen, progesterone).**
  - During puberty, testosterone increases in boys and they gain muscle and lose fat. Men with low testosterone lose fat and gain muscle when testosterone is replaced. Testosterone is important for weight gain/loss.
  - During puberty, estrogen increases, and girls gain body fat in the breasts and hips. Increasing the sex hormone progesterone (with drugs like megestrol) increases appetite and weight. Sex hormones are important for weight gain/loss.

33

- **Thyroid hormones.** Patients with excessively high thyroid levels lose weight. Patients with excessively low thyroid levels gain weight. Therefore, thyroid function is important for weight gain/loss.
- **Brain reward pathways (dopamine, serotonin).** If we interfere with the brain reward pathways (with drugs like antipsychotic or antidepressant medications), people gain weight. If we block these pathways (with drugs like naltrexone/bupropion (Contrave)), people lose weight. Therefore, the brain reward pathways (neurotransmitters) are important for weight gain/loss.

Does this simple causal test work for calories? The answer, backed by decades of experimental research, is ... hell no. Overfeeding calories, such as Drs. Bray and Sims rediscovered in their famous experiments, doesn't cause long-term weight gain. Reducing calories, tested by millions of people and many studies, doesn't cause long-term weight loss.

The nerves and hormones don't directly affect calories, just as the room thermostat does not directly heat or cool the room. When you adjust the room thermostat up or down, it activates the heating or cooling system so that the room temperature matches the new setting. In your body, the nerves and hormones move the body fat thermostat up or down, which changes factors such as hunger, satiety, body heat generation, and metabolic rate. This change causes the weight gain or weight loss needed to match the new body fat thermostat setting. This is the deeper understanding of mechanisms of weight gain or loss, rather than the shallow, superficial notion of Calories In, Calories Out.

In Chapter 4, we will discuss these neurohormonal systems and also some hormones that don't quite meet the standard of causal factors yet may still play an important role in eating behavior. These hormones include

34

- **ghrelin,** the hormone that stimulates appetite, and
- **satiety hormones** (peptide YY, cholecystokinin), hormones that signal fullness, which suppresses appetite.

> **Tip #4:** Focus on the neurohormonal factors to lose weight.
> Obesity is a hormonal rather than a caloric imbalance
> and different foods affect hormones differently.

HOW FOOD AFFECTS HORMONES

DIFFERENT FOODS STIMULATE different hormones. This is a scientifically well-established fact. It is not controversial. It is easily measurable. If you eat white bread, your blood glucose and the hormone insulin go up, too. If you eat an egg, blood glucose and insulin do *not* go up. Our body responds differently to the different hormone levels, including how many calories are stored (as body fat). Why would we ever expect different?

- Some foods stimulate insulin. Some don't. This matters.
- Some foods stimulate glucagon-like peptide 1 (GLP-1). Some don't. This matters.
- Some foods stimulate glucose-dependent insulinotropic polypeptide (GIP). Some don't. This matters.
- Some foods stimulate sympathetic tone. Some don't. This matters.
- Some foods fill up the stomach. Some don't. This matters.
- Some foods stimulate brain reward pathways like dopamine. Some don't. This matters.

Practically speaking, what this really means is **that some foods are more fattening than other foods**. This fact seems like pure common sense. Cookies are more fattening than broccoli, even if you eat the same number of calories. Cookies provoke hormones that cause more of those calories to be stored. It's scientific fact. "Experts" tell you that "a calorie is a calorie," but **all calories are not equally fattening**.

Hormones affect weight gain/loss. Different foods affect hormones differently. This effect depends on many factors, which we'll discuss further, including

35

- the amount of food consumed,
- the macronutrient composition of the food,
- the food matrix,
- the level of processing of the food,
- the Glycemic Index/glycemic load of the food,
- the amount of fiber in the food,
- the volume (bulkiness) of the food,
- the speed of digestion of the food,
- the speed of absorption of the food,
- the order in which you eat each food, and
- the timing of your meals.

The hormonal obesity theory is a nuanced, multifactorial view that places obesity within the framework of normal human physiology. When we understand that many neurohormonal factors contribute to whether we gain or lose weight, we can design a full suite of tools to address the problem. We can also better understand why shoehorning the simplistic, failed notion that "a calorie is a calorie" into the framework of a complex multifaceted disease like obesity is futile.

Not every case of weight gain has the same root cause, and therefore no one solution will work for everyone. When we understand the reason for the weight gain, we can design the appropriate solution. For one person, the root cause of weight gain may be emotional eating; for another, eating ultra-processed foods. The causes are different, and therefore the treatments are different too.

Essentially, to successfully lose weight and keep it off, we need to understand that there are good calories and there are bad calories. The key to regulating the body fat thermostat is regulating our nerves and hormones, and we can do that by eating foods that contain good calories rather than bad ones. Just ask your grandmother. She would have told you the truth.

EATING A
LOW-INSULIN DIET

R EFINED CARBOHYDRATES ARE the bell-bottom jeans of the nutrition world: they were great in the 1970s and terrible in the 2020s. The *Dietary Goals for the United States* released in 1977 (and renamed *Dietary Guidelines for Americans* in 1980) provide direction on what to eat and drink to meet nutrient needs, promote health, and prevent disease. It turns out that these guidelines are more fashion than science. In 1977, commercial white bread was considered healthy because it is low in fat. By the 2020s, the very same white bread is considered unhealthy as a highly refined carbohydrate. In 1977, fatty foods like nuts, fatty fish, and avocados were deemed unhealthy. Dietary fat causes heart disease, don't you know? By the 2020s, the very same nuts, fatty fish, and avocados are considered good-for-you "superfoods." Healthy fats prevent heart disease, don't you know?

Like those bell-bottoms, the dietary advice rooted in the 1970s did not age well and brought unintended consequences. The *Dietary Guidelines* fixated on nutrients (fat, protein, calories) rather than on foods (cabbage, beef, eggs). This reductionist thinking imagines that all nutrients are the same. A calorie is a calorie, whether from cookies or broccoli. All carbohydrates are the same, whether from sugary cereal or bean salad. This thinking is absurd, although repeated often enough, it started to seem reasonable. Imagine saying that all human beings are mostly carbon and so is charcoal, and so replacing Brad Pitt with a lump of charcoal is roughly the same. All calories are not the same. All carbohydrates are not the same. All fats are not the same. Brad Pitt is not a lump of charcoal.

Eating all those refined carbs spiked the glycemic load, a measure of blood glucose, of the average American diet by a massive 22 percent.[1] Blood glucose is the primary form of energy from carbohydrates. More refined carbs means higher blood glucose, which triggers the body to produce insulin. Remember, it's the hormone insulin that directs the body to release or store energy calories. Higher insulin means more weight gain. The upsurge in obesity tracked the increase in carbohydrate consumption—from roughly 375 grams/day in 1960 to more than 500 grams/day by 1997—almost perfectly (Figure 3.1[2]).[3]

Figure 3.1. Increase in obesity in the U.S. between 1960 and 1997

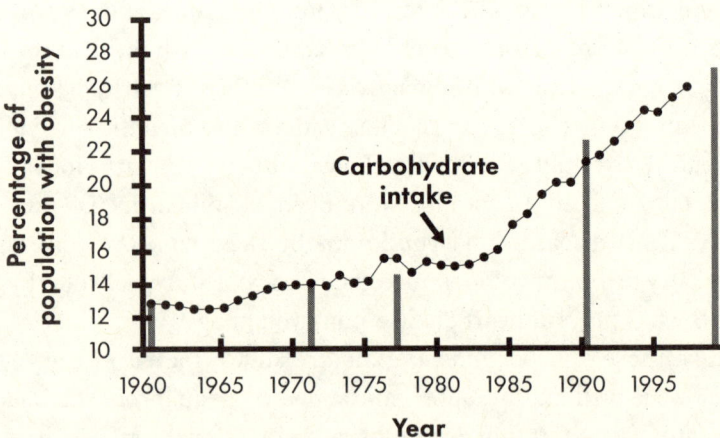

GLUCOSE, INSULIN, AND THE CONNECTION
BETWEEN CARBOHYDRATES AND WEIGHT GAIN

PLANTS STORE EXCESS ENERGY from photosynthesis in the form of carbohydrates, and animals store their excess energy from food as fat. This reality explains why plant-heavy diets typically contain more carbohydrates, which stimulate the greatest insulin surge. Eating fewer total carbohydrates can certainly reduce insulin levels, but that is not the only way. Many traditional diets are based on carbohydrates, and yet people eating those carbohydrate-heavy diets still avoided obesity for generations. The Irish and Germans have traditionally loved their potatoes. The Asians have traditionally loved their rice. The Italians have loved their pasta. The key is to lower **insulin** levels, which is not necessarily the same as eating fewer carbohydrates.

Carbohydrates are sugar. There are many types of sugar, which can be easily identified since they usually end in the suffix *-ose*. Common sugars include glucose, fructose, lactose, and sucrose (table sugar). The main sugar in the human diet and in the human body is glucose. Blood glucose is also known as blood sugar. Starches (wheat, rice, oats, and so on) are long chains of glucose arranged in a structure comprising amylopectin (about 70%) and amylose (about 30%) (Figure 3.2).

Figure 3.2. The way their glucose molecules are arranged differentiates the starches amylose and amylopectin

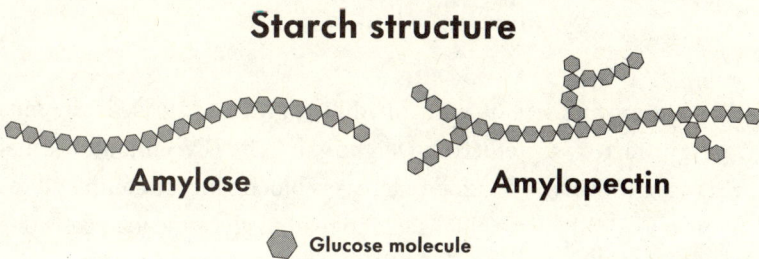

Starch structure

Amylose   **Amylopectin**

⬡ Glucose molecule

Carbohydrates used to be classified as simple carbohydrates if they contained two or fewer sugars in a chain (for example, sucrose) and complex carbohydrates (for example, starches) if they were longer chains. This classification was based on the incorrect assumption that complex carbohydrates are digested and absorbed slowly and that simple carbohydrates are digested and absorbed quickly. But this classification is as useless as a wet newspaper. For example, white bread, a "complex carbohydrate," spikes blood glucose higher and faster than table sugar. We now classify starches by physiology, or how quickly blood glucose rises after eating them (Table 3.1), rather than their chemical structure.

Table 3.1. Modern classification of starches, by timing of glucose release

Type of starch	Timing of glucose release after eating	Effect on the body	Example
Rapidly digestible starch (RDS)	Within 20 minutes	Bad	Commercial white bread
Slowly digestible starch (SDS)	Within 20 to 120 minutes	Better	Steel cut oats
Resistant starch (RS)	No glucose is released (not digested)	Best	Chia seeds

The timing and size of a carbohydrate's glucose release is the most important factor in predicting weight gain. The Glycemic Index measures the speed at which a food increases blood glucose compared to a reference food (like pure glucose). The related glycemic load considers both the Glycemic Index and the amount of carbohydrate in a serving, which provides a more realistic picture of how much the food is affecting blood sugar. Both Glycemic Index and glycemic load are measured on a scale of 0 to 100. A higher Glycemic Index means that blood glucose rises higher and more quickly, which causes higher insulin levels. The higher the insulin, the more weight is gained. The total number of carbohydrates is an important factor in weight gain, but how quickly blood glucose spikes is also critical. This rate depends on the speed at which the food is digested and absorbed.

The standard paradigm of metabolism suggests that we eat food, which contains calories and other macronutrients, which leads to weight gain (Figure 3.3).

Figure 3.3. We have long believed that eating calories leads directly to weight gain

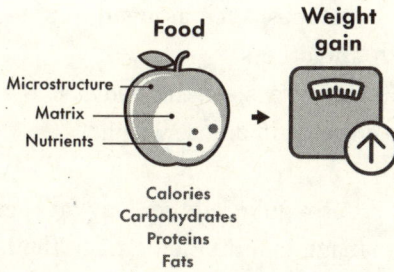

This understanding is woefully deficient, because it completely ignores the effects of digestion, absorption, and hormones. Each step along the metabolic pathway can influence weight gain (Figure 3.4). Understanding the process of weight gain better means that we can devise better treatments. A more comprehensive and correct physiological sequence from food to metabolism looks like this:

Figure 3.4. The path from eating to storing body fat comprises several intermediate steps

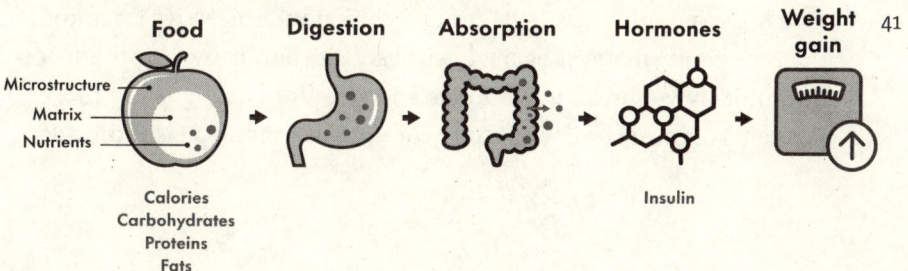

1. **Food:** What we eat contains macronutrients such as carbohydrates, proteins, and fats. We measure total food energy in calories.
2. **Digestion:** Before we can use food for energy, repair, or growth, it must be broken down into smaller, simpler nutrients. Digestion is this process of making food easier for the body to absorb and can include mechanical or enzymatic methods such as refining, cooking, chewing, blending, and churning by the stomach.
3. **Absorption:** The energy and nutrients of the food are absorbed by cells in the intestines and passed into the bloodstream. Processes like cooking, grinding, blending, and refining foods affect how quickly the body absorbs these nutrients.
4. **Hormones:** The presence of different nutrients in the blood triggers different hormones, such as insulin, GLP-1, GIP, peptide YY, cholecystokinin, and others.
5. **Weight gain:** Hormones set the body fat thermostat and give instructions to either gain or lose weight.

When we talk about regulating the body fat thermostat, we know that we need to manage insulin. Remember, the higher the insulin level in the body, the more body fat will be deposited. However, we now understand that to reduce insulin in the body, we need to think not only about what foods we eat but also about how quickly those foods will be digested and absorbed. Both of those processes are important for determining how quickly blood glucose is absorbed and therefore how much insulin is triggered and how quickly.

HOW THE SPEED OF DIGESTION AFFECTS INSULIN RELEASE

DIGESTION MAY SEEM like a simple, straightforward process. We put food in our mouth, chew it, let it move through the digestive tract, and then poop out whatever hasn't been absorbed. But many factors affect how quickly we break down foods and therefore how quickly those nutrients are absorbed. We need to consider whether food is processed, what size the processed particles are, and how quickly they raise blood glucose (Glycemic Index). We also need to think about how much amylose, fiber, and resistant starch each food contains. And finally, we need to think about the way the nutrients are arranged in the food (its food matrix) and its beta-glucans. All of these influence the speed of digestion.

Although digestion begins in the mouth, the stomach not only mechanically churns the food and mixes it with stomach acid, but it also acts as a reservoir. Since we eat food faster than we can absorb its nutrients, the stomach holds the digested food and releases nutrients into the small intestine a little at a time. From there, the nutrients get absorbed into the bloodstream.

We know that carbohydrates break down into glucose, and glucose triggers insulin. So carbohydrates can lead to more weight gain than other macronutrients. But just as not all calories are equal, neither are all carbohydrates equal when it comes to digestion. The enzymes that digest starches and glucose are called amylases, and anything that makes it easier for the amylases to break down these carbs will spike blood glucose. Here are some attributes of food to consider.

Food processing and particle size

Natural carbohydrates are often contained within a physical barrier that resists digestion, such as an intact plant cell wall (whole grains, steel cut oats). They also commonly contain an indigestible type of carbohydrate, fiber. For example, rice is naturally covered by a tough outer husk. Whole-wheat grains are protected by a tough outer shell of bran. The intact plant cell wall, large particle size, and presence of fiber slow digestion significantly. Blood glucose rises more slowly and therefore insulin levels also rise more slowly. Less insulin means less weight gain.

In contrast, refined carbohydrates are digested and absorbed much, much more quickly and easily than natural carbohydrates. When wheat is refined, the bran, germ, and oils that all slow digestion are removed. Then the particles are machine-ground into a very fine dust (flour) that requires no chewing (Figure 3.5[4]). Similarly, when rice is milled, the

43

husk and inner bran are removed. The remaining starchy seed is polished into white rice.

Figure 3.5. What's lost when wheat is refined

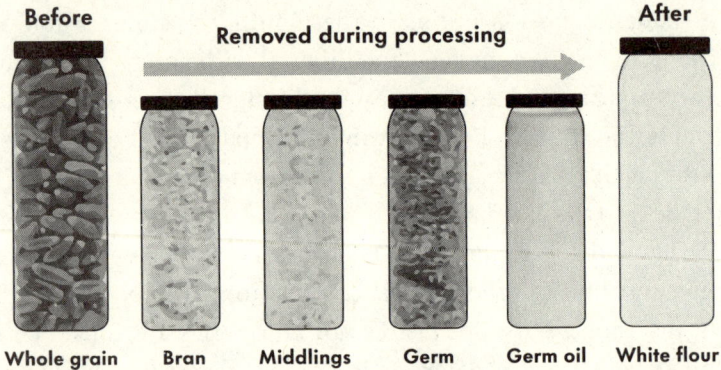

Refining essentially "pre-digests" the carbohydrates, turning them into rapidly digestible starches. Chewing and churning in the stomach helps the amylases rapidly break down the long glucose chains into single glucose molecules that are quickly absorbed. When food particles are smaller and softer, the amylases act faster and therefore the stomach empties faster. If the stomach empties quickly, this very quick absorption of glucose leads to a massive spike in blood glucose and a massive spike in insulin. More insulin means more weight gain.

> **Tip #5:** Eat fewer refined (starchy) carbohydrates.

A recent large study revealed that refined grains and starchy vegetables like bread, rice, and potatoes were associated with a 2.6 kg (5.7 pound) weight gain over four years.[5] In contrast, eating *non-starchy* carbohydrates like broccoli, cabbage, and zucchini was associated with a 3 kg (6.6 pound) weight *loss*. The type of carbohydrate (natural versus refined and processed) makes a big difference. Grandma was right: you should eat your veggies (and french fries are still not a vegetable).

Foods that don't contain carbohydrates generally have a Glycemic Index and glycemic load of zero. It's quite simple, really: carbohydrates are glucose. If you eat glucose, your blood glucose goes up. If you eat proteins and fats, which don't have glucose, then your blood glucose does *not* go up.

Fast versus slow carbs (Glycemic Index)

How quickly carbohydrates are digested and absorbed makes a huge difference to the body's blood glucose levels, and this difference can be measured by the Glycemic Index. Consider three different breakfasts with identical calories:

1. Low Glycemic Index breakfast: Vegetable omelet (40% carbs)
2. Medium Glycemic Index breakfast: Steel cut oatmeal (64% carbs)
3. High Glycemic Index breakfast: Instant oatmeal (64% carbs)

The vegetable omelet contains fewer carbohydrates than the other two options. Based on this information alone, we expect this breakfast to raise blood glucose less than the oatmeal breakfasts, and we are right.

What about the oat breakfasts? The oatmeal in both contains the same number of calories and carbohydrates. They are even the same food. However, steel cut oats are natural carbohydrates that preserve the cell wall of the oat kernel, making digestion very slow. Instant oats are pre-digested, refined carbohydrates that have been pulverized to a fine dust for quick cooking. Instant oats are rapidly digested, and the glucose is absorbed quickly.

The only difference between steel cut and instant oats is the level of processing. Does this matter? Oh, yes. In a study measuring the Glycemic Index of these three breakfasts, the total glucose effect of the instant oats was almost *four times* higher than the omelet, and *almost double* that of the steel cut oats. And there's more bad news. After breakfast, the group that ate the instant oats subsequently ate *81 percent* more calories at the next meal compared to the group that ate the omelet and *53 percent* more calories than the group that ate the steel cut oats. Ouch.

45

Intuitively, you already knew that eggs are more satiating than instant oats. Eat a vegetable omelet for breakfast, and you're full until lunch. Eat highly refined carbohydrates and you're hungry by mid-morning. The difference is not the calories, which were identical, or even the carbohydrates. It's the speed at which those carbs are digested.

Eating fewer carbohydrates improves blood glucose, as expected. But the speed that nutrients are digested and absorbed is also critical. Highly refined carbohydrates elicit a high Glycemic Index and high insulin response compared to less-processed carbohydrates, which leads to eating more afterward.[6] In a similar study, kids who ate cornflakes and bananas (high glycemic load) versus eggs and strawberries (low glycemic load) for breakfast ate 65 *percent* more calories at lunchtime. Despite equal-calorie breakfasts, they ate almost two-thirds more at lunch![7]

Consider the effect from your body's point of view. The breakfast of "pre-digested" instant oats massively spikes glucose and insulin, which orders your body to store the calories. The strength of the insulin spike pushes most of the glucose (and calories) into storage (body fat), leaving you little energy for basic metabolic processes like generating body heat and powering your brain, heart, liver, kidneys, and other vital organs. About two hours after you eat the instant oats, your blood glucose crashes, and you become hypoglycemic. To counter this abnormal decrease in blood glucose, your body sends out hunger signals, and you go out looking for more food. With the omelet breakfast, insulin doesn't go up much, so fewer calories are stored (body fat), leaving most of them available for metabolism. You stay fuller for longer and eat less at the next meal. It's not magic; it all makes perfect physiological sense.

Try to keep the carbs in your diet as natural and unprocessed as possible. When choosing bread, look for stone-ground flour, which leaves particles larger than machine-ground flour and slows digestion. Both pumpernickel (Glycemic Index 45) and rye (Glycemic Index 65) bread have a lower glycemic load than white bread (95). Rye flour is high in fiber, and traditional pumpernickel is made with coarsely ground rye flour with a sourdough starter. The fermentation process of sourdough generates lactic acid, which reduces the glucose effect.

46

> **Tip #6:** Choose foods with a low Glycemic Index
> and glycemic load and avoid rapidly digested starches.

> **Tip #7:** Keep carbohydrates as natural and unprocessed as possible. Prefer coarsely ground (stone-ground) rather than finely ground (machine-ground) flour due to its larger particle size.

Branched (amylopectin) versus linear (amylose) starches

The prefix *amyl-* is derived from the Greek word for "mill" and refers to starches. The chains of glucose that form starches can be highly branched (amylopectin) or arranged in a linear helix (amylose). Amylopectin is easily dissolved in water, which makes it easier to digest. So foods high in amylopectin are rapidly digested and absorbed, and spike blood glucose and insulin. In contrast, the compact packing and layered crystalline structure of amylose makes it harder to digest, and so the glucose is released more slowly, lowering its insulin effect.[8]

So which foods contain which kind of starch? This question is particularly important when it comes to rice, which is eaten by over two-thirds of the world's population. Different types of rice contain different concentrations of amylopectin and amylose.[9] After rice is harvested, the husk is removed, leaving brown rice. This brown rice is often polished to make it white, which removes the bran with its oils, vitamins, and minerals. Rice varieties that are sticky when cooked—like short-grain, sticky, and glutinous rice—are very high in amylopectin and contain little to no amylose. They increase blood glucose quickly. Sticky rice, for example, has the highest Glycemic Index at 98. Rice varieties that are fluffy when cooked—like jasmine and basmati—contain a higher amount of amylose (25–30%). They are slower to digest and typically have a Glycemic Index of around 58. Converted, or parboiled rice, which is partially cooked with the husk on and then cooled, is slow to digest because it contains the whole grain. Converted rice causes blood glucose to rise very gradually and has the lowest Glycemic Index (38).[10]

47

Foods that are high in amylose include quinoa, beans, lentils, and oats. Arrowroot powder, which is used for thickening, contains almost 30 percent amylose and may be a better choice than cornstarch. Baby potatoes have higher levels of amylose compared to regular potatoes, so they may be a better choice, though the difference is slight.

If you're going to eat foods containing amylopectin, you'll want to know the differences between A, B, and C chains. Amylopectin A is the most easily digestible. Products made from wheat contain mostly type A and cause blood glucose to rise quickly. Amylopectin B is moderately digestible, and these chains are found in potatoes and bananas. Beans are a good source of amylopectin C, which is the hardest to digest. The undigested starch is not absorbed, and so it is delivered to the colon, where it ferments. The fermentation causes gas and commonly triggers flatulence (farts) and hysterical laughter from adolescent boys, and most grown men, too.

> **Tip #8:** Choose amylose starches like quinoa,
> lentils, baby potatoes, oats, and beans.

Fiber and resistant starch

Both dietary fiber and resistant starches are carbohydrates that cannot be digested, so no glucose is absorbed, and blood glucose and insulin don't go up. No insulin means no fat storage and no weight gain.

Fiber is a non-starch polysaccharide found in the cell wall of plants. Fiber increases the bulk of the food, which stretches the stomach and makes you feel full. In the colon, the fiber is fermented to short-chain fatty acids (SCFAs) such as acetate, butyrate, and propionate. These SCFAs increase satiety hormones such as GLP-1 and peptide YY.[11]

Good sources of fermentable fiber include apples, almonds, avocados, pears, cabbage, Brussels sprouts, carrots, grapefruit, whole oats, beans, lentils, peas, chickpeas, chia seeds, and oranges. Chia seeds can be added to many drinks without affecting the taste. They form a viscous layer that partially blocks glucose absorption and increases satiety.

ALL ABOUT OATS

Steel cut oats, also called Irish oats, are whole oat kernels cut with steel blades into pieces the size of two or three pinheads. They have lots of fiber and are minimally processed, so they must be cooked for approximately forty minutes with plenty of liquid to be edible. Even then, steel cut oats are digested very slowly, which means they have the lowest insulin effect.

The most popular oats are rolled oats, which have a Glycemic Index higher than steel cut oats, but lower than instant. Rolled oats are steamed, flattened between rollers, and then dried in a kiln, which increases the amylose content. Thicker oats are more slowly digested. Thinner oats, sometimes called "quick oats" are more easily digested, and therefore have a higher Glycemic Index.

Instant ("quick") oatmeal is steamed longer, flattened more, and then ground into the tiniest of pieces, allowing them to be cooked in under two minutes, usually just by adding hot water. This processing means these "predigested" oats are quickly absorbed and therefore have a high Glycemic Index. Quick digestion = Blood glucose spike = More insulin = More weight gain.

Beta-glucans are a type of soluble fiber that occurs naturally in some grains, including oats, barley, and rye, and in some types of mushrooms. When dissolved in water, beta-glucans form a viscous, gel-like substance. So, although oats are high in carbohydrates, they are relatively high in protein (14%) compared to other grains, contain 25 to 30 percent amylose (which can bind with fats to form resistant starch), and contain significant (4%) beta-glucans. The higher viscosity reduces the rate of digestion, stomach emptying, and glucose release.[12] Slower digestion means lower insulin means less weight gain.

49

Oat bran is made from grinding oat grain and separating out the bran. It has 5.5 percent beta-glucans and lots of dietary fiber. Adding oat bran to foods can significantly reduce their Glycemic Index due to its high dietary fiber.

Tip #9: Eat more fiber to satisfy hunger and keep insulin low.

Tip #10: Eat steel cut oats, not instant,
for their high-soluble fiber.

Resistant starches are chains of glucose molecules that cannot be digested. Some of these starches are naturally indigestible (native resistant starches), but you can increase the resistant starch in some foods like rice by cooking and then cooling them (retrograded resistant starches). Cooking rice causes the starches to become more liquid (gelatinize) and, when cooled, the liquid starch forms a new crystal structure (retrogradation). That's why cold rice is brittle and hard to eat. When cold rice is reheated, some of the retrograded resistant starches remain and the partially crystallized structure is more difficult for our digestive enzyme amylase to break down. This effect slows down digestion and the rate at which our stomach empties, which makes us feel more full. Blood glucose also does not spike, which keeps the Glycemic Index low and decreases the glucose and insulin effect.[13]

Cooking, refrigerating, and then reheating rice increases the resistant starch by almost two-and-a-half times.[14] The resistant starches increase the longer the rice is cooled, even up to seven days.[15] When reheated, the higher proportion of resistant starch reduces the glycemic effect. In Asian cuisine, fried rice usually is made by cooking and cooling rice before frying.

This process doesn't work for potatoes. Cooking, refrigerating, and then reheating does not increase the resistant starch because the retrogradation that took place during cooking and cooling is reversed while reheating. To maximize resistant starches in potatoes, eat them cold, when their resistant starch content is increased by 57 percent. A cold potato salad with vinegar reduces the Glycemic Index by 43 percent and insulin by 31 percent compared to hot potatoes.[16] Less insulin means less weight gain.

> **Tip #11:** Eat more resistant starches. Cook, cool, and reheat rice. Eat cooked potatoes cold.

The food matrix

The food matrix is the physical structure in which a food's nutrients are embedded. Think of it as the packaging. Suppose you give your friend a gift, like a mug. You could give them the mug by itself, but putting it in a fancy box with a nice ribbon and a gift bag changes its perceived value. Similarly, two foods may have identical nutrients, but when they are arranged differently, by cooking, grinding, refining, and so on, their physiological effect is changed.

The way the nutrients are arranged in the food—the food matrix—affects the speed of digestion and therefore the Glycemic Index. For example, pasta (Glycemic Index 50) and white bread (Glycemic Index 75) are both made from flour, a highly refined carbohydrate, but their Glycemic Index is very different. Why? In cooked pasta, the starch granules (carbohydrates) are mixed with the main protein, gluten. The starch granules gelatinize as they cook and then thicken into a mass (coagulate) with the glutens (protein network), making the pasta harder to digest. This slower digestion lessens the glucose and insulin effect by about 40 percent compared to white bread, whose food matrix is more porous and therefore easier and quicker to digest.[17] Slower digestion means lower Glycemic Index means less insulin means less weight gain. That's good.

Like pasta, parboiled rice with tomato sauce has a lower Glycemic Index than white bread. The rice and tomato sauce have a peak insulin effect that's about 45 percent lower than the insulin effect of

51

commercial white bread.[18] Why? The amylose (starch) in the rice binds with the fats in the tomato sauce to form a type of resistant starch known as an amylose-lipid complex. Essentially, the fats fill in the gaps in the starch's helical structure, making it heat stable to about 212 degrees Fahrenheit (100 degrees Celsius) and hard to digest. This food matrix results in slower digestion, which reduces insulin. Less insulin means less weight gain.

Tip #12: Choose pasta and low-glycemic rice over white bread.

Eating calories or nutrients doesn't cause weight gain directly. The foods must first be digested, which prepares the nutrients for absorption into the bloodstream, which influences the hormonal response, which dictates whether we gain weight. Many, many factors influence the speed of digestion, which ultimately impacts the insulin response (Figure 3.6).

Figure 3.6. Many factors influence the speed of digestion, and quick digestion increases insulin

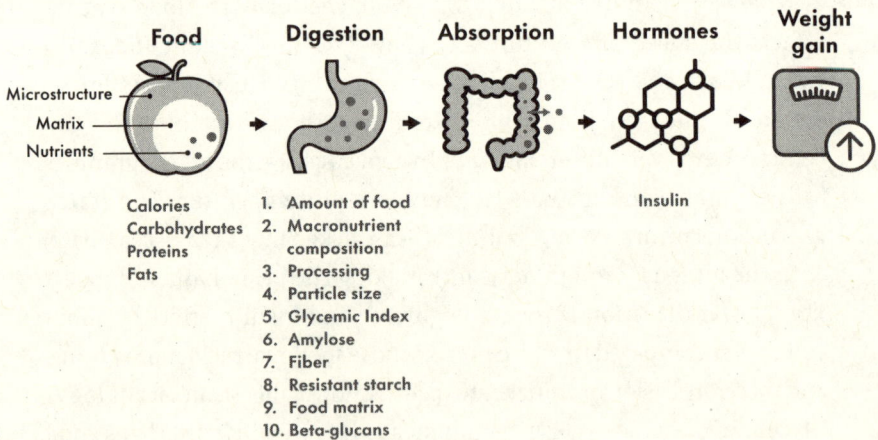

Food	Digestion	Absorption	Hormones	Weight gain

Microstructure
Matrix
Nutrients

Calories
Carbohydrates
Proteins
Fats

1. Amount of food
2. Macronutrient composition
3. Processing
4. Particle size
5. Glycemic Index
6. Amylose
7. Fiber
8. Resistant starch
9. Food matrix
10. Beta-glucans

Insulin

HOW THE SPEED OF ABSORPTION
AFFECTS INSULIN RELEASE

BREAKING FOOD DOWN into its individual nutrients—digestion—is a key first step in providing the body with energy. Next, those nutrients must get into the bloodstream so they can enter the cells. That's primarily the job of the small intestine through the process of absorption. As we've seen, foods that are quickly digested are also often quickly absorbed, so many of the factors that contribute to fast or slow digestion are also important for absorption. However, the bulkiness of the foods, the way they are prepared, and their viscosity and acidity play a larger role in how quickly they are absorbed. Also important is how the foods are served, including naked or dressed, in what order, and at what time. All of these factors have an effect on the speed of absorption.

The rate of gastric emptying

How quickly food is released from the stomach after digestion—gastric emptying—is an important factor in absorption. The stomach mixes the foods we eat with stomach acid, churns the mixture, and releases it in a measured fashion into the intestines where the nutrients are absorbed. If nutrients are released quickly, then the speed of absorption increases. If nutrients are delayed in the stomach, then the speed of absorption must slow since no nutrients cross the stomach into the bloodstream. The faster nutrients are absorbed, the higher the glucose spike and the more insulin is produced. This effect depends on many factors, none of which can be found alongside the information about nutrients such as calories, carbohydrates, fats, and proteins on any food label.

Food preparation (cooking, puréeing, juicing, blending)

Different methods of preparing foods change both their digestibility and their absorption, which changes their hormonal effect. For example, consider equal calorie portions of whole apple slices, applesauce (cooked and blended apples), and apple juice (juiced apples). Each of these apple servings produces dramatically different physiological effects.[19]

Pre-digested foods are absorbed more quickly. In one study, participants who ate 125 calories of whole apple slices at one meal subsequently ate 312 fewer calories at the next meal. In comparison, participants who ate applesauce (125 calories) at the first meal ate 221 fewer calories at the next meal. And those who drank apple juice (125 calories) at the first meal ate only 125 fewer calories at the next meal. Why? The stomach holds the whole apples longer, which keeps us feeling fuller, and therefore we eat less later on. The time required for the stomach to empty by half is sixty-five minutes for apple slices, forty-one minutes for applesauce, and thirty-eight minutes for juice.[20] Cooking the apples (applesauce) and juicing the apples (apple juice) pre-digests the nutrients so the stomach releases them more quickly for absorption. Quicker absorption means higher blood glucose, higher insulin, and more weight gain.

> **Tip #13:** Eat whole fruits, not cooked, puréed, or juiced fruits.

Surprisingly, blending fruits, like in a smoothie, can be a useful way to slow the absorption of nutrients for seeded fruits. The dietary fiber, proteins, fats, and polyphenols contained within the seeds are released during blending, which increases the viscosity of the fruit and slows the rate of gastric emptying. Slower absorption means lower blood glucose, which means less insulin and less weight gain.

Raspberry, strawberry, and passion-fruit seeds are particularly high in polyphenols, which inhibit pancreatic amylases, further slowing glucose absorption.[21] In one study, blending a mango with raspberries and passion fruit significantly reduced the glucose (and therefore the insulin) response.[22] Similarly, an apple and blackberry smoothie has about one-third less of the glucose effect of whole apples and blackberries.[23]

> **Tip #14:** Blend seeded fruits into smoothies
> to release their fiber and other nutrients.

Fructose is fruit sugar. In *The Obesity Code*, we described how fructose is metabolized differently from glucose and actually causes more insulin resistance. So can you eat fruit? Small amounts of fructose, like the amounts found in whole fruit, can be metabolized by the cells of the small intestine into glucose. It's the larger amounts found in ultra-processed foods that overwhelm the small intestine and are mostly diverted to the liver. Too much fructose accumulating in the liver causes fatty liver.[24] As much as possible, minimize fruits that are high in fructose, such as mangoes, grapes, and watermelon. Instead, choose lower-fructose fruits, such as berries, kiwis, and non-sweet fruits like coconuts, avocados, and olives.

Tip #15: Choose lower-fructose fruits like berries and avoid higher-fructose fruits like grapes, mangoes, and watermelon.

Food viscosity

Viscosity describes the thickness or stickiness of a liquid. Our brain perceives thicker liquids as more food-like, which stimulates GLP-1, a known satiety hormone, and reduces hunger by as much as 30 percent.[25] Drinks that are thicker reduce hunger better, even when calories, fiber, and sugar are the same.[26] And drinking soups with a thicker, more viscous consistency fills the stomach with a gel-like matrix that slows gastric emptying and makes us feel full.[27]

Viscous foods help slow the speed of absorption in two ways. First, they stimulate hormones that make us feel full, so we eat less. When we eat less, we have fewer nutrients to absorb. One study found that eating semi-solids like yogurt, jelly, or sour cream reduces future food intake by 99 calories.[28] Viscous fluids like soup feel like part of the meal, so you'll eat less subsequently. Second, viscous foods take longer to digest, which means the stomach releases them more slowly into the intestine for absorption. Increasing viscosity by adding chia seeds to liquids creates a gel-like matrix that slows digestion and absorption.

> **Tip #16:** Drink thicker, slower-digesting liquids like soup.
> Add chia seeds for viscosity and fiber.

Acidic foods

To digest carbohydrates, we rely on enzymes called amylases in the saliva and the pancreas. Salivary amylases do about 65 to 80 percent of the work of breaking the long glucose chains of starchy foods into individual glucose molecules. Acidic foods, including lemon juice (citric acid) and vinegar (acetic acid), as well as fermented foods (lactic acid) help to block these salivary amylases, which slows digestion. Pancreatic amylases in the small intestine finish the job of breaking down glucose so that it can be absorbed.

Eating carbohydrates with organic acids—for example, bread with vinegar (and olive oil) or noodles with kimchi—slows digestion, which means glucose is absorbed more slowly and the insulin effect is reduced by up to 50 percent. One study found that eating bread with vinegar reduced glucose and insulin spike, and people felt more full compared to eating bread alone.[29] Another study found that sushi rice, with its added vinegar, reduced Glycemic Index from 100 to 67, and eating pickled vegetables with rice reduced Glycemic Index by about 25 percent.[30] Lemon juice reduces glucose availability by as much as 35 percent.[31] Lower blood glucose means less insulin means less weight gain, which is a good thing.

> **Tip #17:** Eat more acidic foods, including vinegar (pickled foods), fermented foods (sauerkraut, kimchi), and lemon juice.

"Naked" carbs

56

I call refined carbohydrates eaten on their own, without protein or fats, "naked" carbs. Think of breakfast cereal or white toast with jam or cookies, low-fat muffins, donuts, and cakes. Naked carbs are more or less 100 percent pure glucose. We digest carbs on their own very, very quickly. If you eat your carbs naked, then the stomach holds only glucose. When this glucose gets pushed into the intestines, it is rapidly absorbed by the rest of the body. In other words, that 100 percent pure glucose causes a massive spike in blood glucose and insulin. Not good.

Eating carbohydrates with other foods, such as meat, mixes the glucose with the proteins and fats in the stomach so that it contains a mix of macronutrients rather than 100 percent glucose. That mix slows the speed of digestion, releases the nutrients more slowly into the intestine, and blunts the glucose and insulin spike. The slower glucose is absorbed by the body, the lower the insulin spike.

Avoiding naked carbs is similar to the idea that you shouldn't drink alcohol on an empty stomach. Because the alcohol is not mixed with any food in the stomach, it gets absorbed very quickly making you drunk very quickly. In this case, it's the pure carbohydrate rather than pure alcohol that causes problems.

To avoid naked carbs, build your meal around a protein. At breakfast, start with eggs, bacon, or Greek yogurt. At lunch or dinner, pair veggies with hummus (protein) or build your meal around meat or some black beans or chickpeas. And for dessert, try berries with Greek yogurt (protein) and a handful of nuts (fats).

Food combinations can have absorptive as well as nutritional benefits. A study in Japan found that eating starches with other foods—particularly dairy, soy products (miso, natto), and fats—can reduce the glucose effect by 25 to 30 percent.[32,33,34] The whey proteins in milk and the soluble fiber in soybeans slow the rate of digestion, gastric emptying, and absorption. Rice and beans is a classic combination in many traditional cuisines.

Similarly, dietary fat binds to the amylose in starch to form double helices that inhibit amylase. This type of resistant starch lowers the Glycemic Index and slows gastric emptying.[35] Eating bread with butter, for example, reduces blood glucose by about 30 percent compared to eating bread alone.[36]

> **Tip #18:** Always eat your carbs with proteins and fats.
> Don't eat "naked" carbs.

Food order

Be mindful about the order in which you eat your food. When you eat carbohydrates before eating proteins and fats, you are eating "naked" carbs. As we've just seen, naked carbs are more or less 100 percent pure glucose, which the body digests and absorbs very quickly. Blood glucose spikes initially, but then drops below normal a few hours after eating (Figure 3.7[37]). This low blood sugar—hypoglycemia—can drive hunger, overeating, and weight gain.

Figure 3.7. Comparison of blood glucose levels over three hours after eating carbs first, veggies first, and combined veggies and protein first

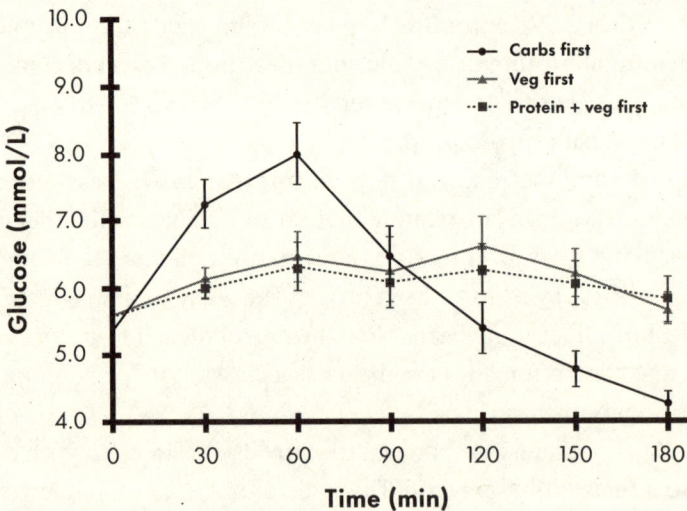

Eating proteins and vegetables before the carbs reduces the glucose and insulin effect by a staggering 40 to 50 percent compared to eating

the carbs first, followed by the protein and vegetables.[38,39] Incredibly, this difference occurs even though the two meals are **identical in every way**, except for the order in which the foods are eaten.

Be especially mindful when eating at restaurants that offer free bread at the start of your meal. First, because you are hungry, you will be tempted to eat more bread than you might otherwise consume. Second, eating these naked carbs first will spike your blood glucose and insulin levels. Third, you'll experience more hunger after the main course. In fact, hypoglycemia often hits just as dessert is being offered. Sugary desserts then cause another blood glucose and insulin spike, and the cycle repeats. Always ask for the bread to be served with or, better yet, after your meal.

> **Tip #19:** Eat carbohydrates last in your meal.

Meal timing

National surveys show that people are eating later and later,[40] and an estimated 65 percent of Americans snack after dinner.[41] Our modern school and working-day schedules, in fact, are built around the late evening meal so that family and friends can gather to eat.

Physiologically, eating late in the day has several notable disadvantages. First, you tend to be hungrier later in the evening. Studies of circadian rhythm show that hunger peaks at about 8 p.m. If you are hungrier, you will likely eat more and eat foods that you know aren't good for you.[42]

Second, you cannot compensate for a large late-evening meal by reducing the size of your other meals. For example, if you eat a big breakfast, you can simply eat less at lunch or dinner. But if you eat a large meal late in the day after two normal meals earlier on, you can't eat less at subsequent meals. The day is over. The deal is done.

Third, eating the same meal at dinner as at breakfast gives you *almost 30 percent more insulin effect*, which tells your body to store more

59

of this food as body fat. Why is food more fattening at night? Our body's circadian rhythm naturally releases certain hormones early in the morning, to prepare for wakefulness and metabolic changes associated with being awake. Growth hormone, which is primarily released during sleep, increases around 5 a.m., as does cortisol, which then decreases throughout the day. Both of these hormones counter insulin.[43]

Even a delay of a few hours makes a difference. Eating the same meal at 6 p.m. instead of 9 p.m. reduces the glucose effect by 30 to 50 percent, and that benefit persists throughout the whole night (Figure 3.8[44]).[45] Eating earlier may result in an extra 4.4 pounds (2 kg) of weight loss over time without extra effort.[46] Eating later lowers the metabolic rate, driving more calories toward fat storage.[47] When you eat earlier, the lower insulin level leaves more food energy (calories) available for metabolism. Eating before bedtime means those calories cannot be used and must therefore be stored (as body fat).

Figure 3.8. Difference in blood glucose levels when eating dinner at 6 p.m. versus 9 p.m.

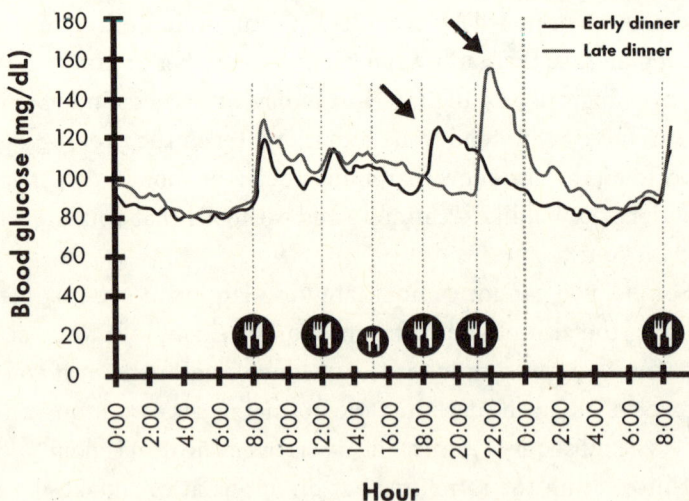

Early time-restricted eating (eTRE, also known as early time-restricted feeding (eTRF)) combines a period of eating early in the day with a lengthy fasting period. This strategy avoids the late, large meal and reduces insulin levels by more than 40 percent (Figure 3.9[48]). Participants who ate earlier also noted much less desire to eat at night, even when asked to.[49,50] Restricting eating to early in the day, rather than skipping breakfast and eating later, can also help to prevent dinnertime from getting too late.

Figure 3.9. Using an early time-restricted eating plan can reduce hunger and increase feelings of fullness, especially in the evening

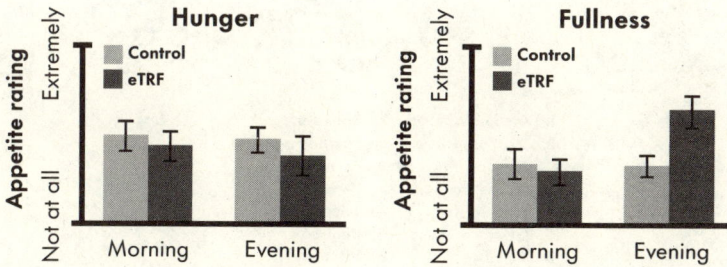

> **Tip #20:** Eat meals earlier in the day, especially meals containing carbs. Avoid large, late dinners and snacks.

To recap, eating late at night increases weight gain because

1. hunger naturally peaks at 8 p.m., so you'll likely eat more. Yikes!
2. hormones that counter insulin peak in the morning, so the foods you eat in the evening will have a more fattening effect. Double yikes!
3. metabolism slows after you eat, so more calories are directed toward storage (as body fat) just as you are heading for a period of rest and inactivity (sleep). Triple yikes!
4. you can't compensate by eating less at a later meal. Quadruple yikes!

HOW TO EAT A LOW-INSULIN DIET

THE HORMONE INSULIN is a key regulator of the body fat thermostat and weight gain. How much insulin is released depends on the macronutrient composition of the meal (fats, proteins, carbohydrates) and the many factors that affect how quickly those nutrients are digested and absorbed (Figure 3.10).

Figure 3.10. Many factors affect how quickly we digest and absorb food, and how much they increase insulin

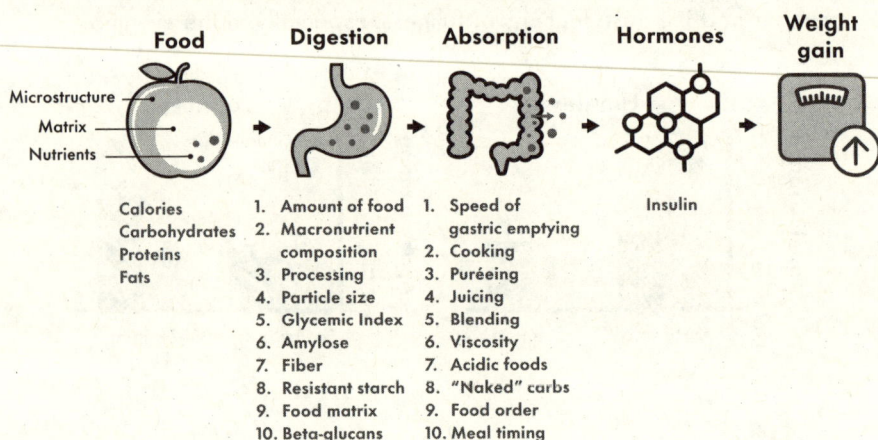

Food	Digestion	Absorption	Hormones	Weight gain
Microstructure Matrix Nutrients				
Calories	1. Amount of food	1. Speed of gastric emptying	Insulin	
Carbohydrates	2. Macronutrient composition	2. Cooking		
Proteins	3. Processing	3. Puréeing		
Fats	4. Particle size	4. Juicing		
	5. Glycemic Index	5. Blending		
	6. Amylose	6. Viscosity		
	7. Fiber	7. Acidic foods		
	8. Resistant starch	8. "Naked" carbs		
	9. Food matrix	9. Food order		
	10. Beta-glucans	10. Meal timing		

Follow these tips to eat a low-insulin diet:

1. Eat fewer refined (starchy) carbohydrates.
2. Choose foods with a low Glycemic Index and glycemic load and avoid rapidly digested starches.
3. Keep carbohydrates as natural and unprocessed as possible. Prefer coarsely ground (stone-ground) rather than finely ground (machine-ground) flour due to its larger particle size.
4. Choose starches with higher amylose or amylopectin C.
5. Eat more fiber.

6. Eat resistant starch.
7. Choose pasta and low-glycemic rice over white bread due to their denser food matrix.
8. Eat steel cut oats instead of instant oats for their high soluble fiber (beta-glucans).
9. Reduce the speed of gastric emptying.
10. Eat whole fruits instead of cooked, puréed, or juiced fruits.
11. Blend seeded fruits into smoothies to release fiber and other nutrients within the seeds.
12. Drink thicker, slower-digesting liquids like soup. Add chia seeds for viscosity and fiber.
13. Eat more acidic foods, including vinegar (pickled foods), fermented foods (sauerkraut, kimchi), and lemon juice.
14. Always eat your carbs with proteins and fats to slow digestion and absorption (don't eat "naked" carbs).
15. Eat carbohydrates last in your meal. Start with proteins and vegetables.
16. Eat meals earlier in the day, especially meals containing carbs. Avoid large, late dinners and snacks.

| 4 |

HOW HORMONES
SUSTAIN HUNGER

IKE THE 2020S, the 2010s bore witness to an immense wave of optimism that obesity was about to be cured. This time, the silver bullet was not a drug; it was weight-loss (bariatric) surgery. For many years, an American reality television show called *My 600-lb Life* has followed people on their journey to reduce their weight to a healthy level. Usually, participants tried to lose weight on their own by following a strict diet, and many were also offered gastric bypass surgery or sleeve gastrectomy. These surgeries reduced the size of the stomach and the volume of nutrients that could be absorbed. The early results were amazing. People lost hundreds of pounds and kept the weight off. For a while. But, in the end, obesity was not cured. Not even close. What happened?

Unfortunately, in the long term, people on the show regained all the weight they'd lost and sometimes even a bit more. The clearest indicator of bariatric surgery's failure was the steadily declining number of surgeries being performed despite the ever-growing epidemic of obesity. The completed number of sleeve gastrectomy operations peaked in 2014, and by 2020 (pre-Covid) had fallen by almost 50 percent.[1] The more powerful Roux-en-Y (gastric bypass) surgery peaked in popularity in 2010, and the number of surgeries has since fallen by over 60 percent. Almost half of the patients who underwent bariatric surgery regretted it.[2]

The issue? Simply, surgery reduced how much food people could physically eat, but it didn't reduce their hunger. The problem was never the calories. The problem was the hunger.

Why do we eat? It's certainly not the calories. Have you ever thought to yourself, "I'm hungry. I should eat 493 calories." Or, "Oh, I ate 462 extra calories at lunch, and so I should only eat 683 calories at dinner." No, doesn't sound familiar. That's why strategies based on calorie counting are completely nonintuitive, non-physiological, and awkward.

On the other hand, tell me if you've ever thought to yourself, "Oh, I'm super hungry. I'm going to order the extra-large burrito." Or, "Oh, I'm so full. I will just have a small salad for dinner." Of course. We have these kinds of thoughts all the time. So we need to acknowledge this fundamental truth:

We eat because we are hungry. We stop eating when we are full.

Homeostatic hunger is driven mainly by neurohormonal factors, as we alluded to in Chapter 2.

Let's explore each of these neurohormonal factors in more detail.

LEPTIN

IN THE MID 1990s, researchers believed they had found the cure for obesity. Fat cells release a protein called leptin. If you have more fat cells, or larger ones, you release more leptin, which tells the appetite centers in the brain (arcuate nucleus) to turn off hunger. This hormone makes you eat less, which reduces insulin and causes weight loss. Your fat cells return to their proper number and size (homeostasis).[3]

Leptin is the signal that "we're too fat." Where insulin turns up the body fat thermostat, leptin turns it down. This negative feedback loop (Figure 4.1) illustrates how the body fat thermostat is supposed to maintain homeostasis of body fat.

Figure 4.1. When insulin turns up the body fat thermostat, leptin is meant to turn it down

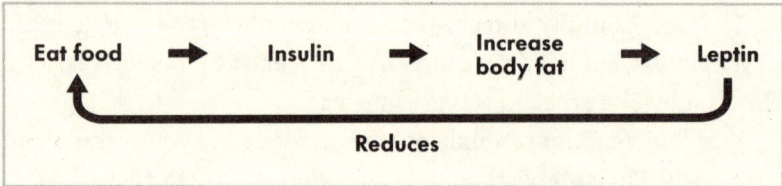

| Eat food | → | Insulin | → | Increase body fat | → | Leptin |

Reduces

Aha, thought the scientists. Obesity is caused by too little leptin. In 1995, the biopharmaceutical company Amgen bought the commercial rights to make synthetic leptin, for a then-record price. Just inject leptin, the thinking went, and then you'll stop eating and lose weight. Why haven't you heard of this miraculous cure? Because for most people, injecting leptin to lose weight didn't work. Leptin levels were not low in overweight people; those levels were already high, and giving more leptin didn't help.

Obesity is a leptin-resistant state. What that means is that although leptin does adjust the body fat thermostat down, it is a weak signal. High insulin levels easily overwhelm leptin, and the thermostat continues to go up. By the time people have gained significant weight, leptin is already as maxed out as the credit card you stupidly let your teenager borrow. Giving more synthetic leptin had no effect.

Leptin explains why Dr. George Bray and other normal-weight people who recently gained weight could so easily lose it. Leptin would shut down their appetite for weeks, until they lost all the weight they'd gained, without any effort or willpower.

GHRELIN AND STOMACH DISTENTION (VAGUS NERVE)

WHEN OUR STOMACH is empty, it secretes the hormone ghrelin, sometimes called the "hunger hormone." This hormone acts on the brain's appetite centers in the hypothalamus to release the hunger-stimulating hormones orexin and melanin-concentrating hormone. You get hungry, so you eat. The food fills the stomach, stretching the receptors in the stomach wall, which are called baroreceptors. Sensing that the stomach is full, the stomach stops secreting ghrelin. This message is transmitted via the vagus nerve to the brain. Together, the baroreceptors and ghrelin turn hunger on and off in a nice, neat homeostatic negative feedback loop (Figure 4.2).

Figure 4.2. Ghrelin turns hunger on and the baroreceptors turn hunger off

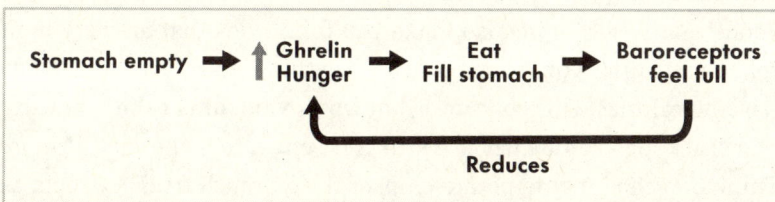

Aha! Maybe obesity is triggered by excessively high ghrelin levels, which cause a "perverted appetite" that leads to overeating and weight gain. This hypothesis, too, is neat, tidy, and plausible—but it is just not correct. Surprisingly, in people with obesity, ghrelin levels are usually lower than normal.[4] As with leptin, ghrelin plays a role in adjusting the body fat thermostat, but a relatively small one. Both hormones lower the body fat thermostat, but by the time you've gained significant weight, these hormones are as exhausted as a snail crawling uphill.

The value of bulky foods

We can use the baroreceptors to help turn down hunger by eating bulky foods that fill up the stomach. Foods that contain more water and fiber, like leafy greens and vegetables, increase the total bulk and therefore produce greater satiety. In addition, foods that are harder, chunkier, more viscous, and/or solid stay in the stomach longer, keeping it more distended and making us fuller for longer.[5] The baroreceptors explain

67

why reducing the rate of stomach emptying benefits satiety, which is useful for weight loss.

The dietary approach to promoting weight loss by filling up on bulky foods is called volumetrics, and it is supported by many clinical studies. People eating the same volume of food felt equally full, whether they ate anywhere from 450 fewer calories[6] to 1430 fewer calories.[7] Eating bulkier foods translates into an additional weight loss of between 1.5 kg (3.3 pounds)[8] and 2.2 kg (4.9 pounds).[9]

The value of heavy foods

Foods that weigh more also make you full. Foods that are very light make you think you are not eating anything and that those foods have no calories. This concept is known as **vanishing caloric density**, and snack food companies use it to great effect to make you eat more. Think of a cheese puff, potato chip, or fluffy french fry. They seem as light as air, and it's easy to just keep eating more. Compare that feeling to a chunk of cheese or a heavy boiled potato. Eating bulky, heavy foods makes us feel full, which keeps hunger at bay.

On a side note, many "experts" advise you to eat "nutrient-dense" foods. I always wonder, "Which nutrients need to be dense?" Have you ever tried to compress a piece of steak? Is squishing vegetables helpful for weight loss? Is getting more vitamin B or C or D in a smaller volume good? Not really. The truth is actually the opposite. Calories are the energy contained within food. To lose weight, you want to eat nutrient-sparse foods: foods with a few nutrients (calories) contained within a large volume. This bulk makes you feel full and helps you maintain an ideal weight. Eating nutrient (calorie) dense donuts is not good. Eating berries, full of water and fiber to increase volume and heft, is much better.

> **Tip #21:** Eat bulky, heavy foods that that contain fiber and water to fill the stomach, such as leafy green vegetables, berries, beans, whole oats, cauliflower, and broccoli.

The value of adequate sleep

Sleep and eating are more related than you might think. Shorter sleep is associated with higher rates of obesity,[10] and a third of American adults report regularly sleeping less than the recommended eight hours per night. Sleep deprivation increases ghrelin, the hunger hormone.[11] Even a single night of sleep deprivation increases ghrelin levels by 22 percent, which caused a doubling in subjective feelings of hunger.[12] Women experienced a higher rise in ghrelin after sleep loss compared to men.[13]

Weight loss depends on controlling hunger. Sleep deprivation increases both the hunger and the opportunity to eat. Go to bed and wake earlier, and schedule an extra half hour of total sleep. Hunger is highest in the evenings, and late-night snacking stimulates more insulin compared to the same foods eaten in the morning. By sleeping earlier (for example, at 10:30 p.m. instead of 11 p.m.), you minimize the time spent in a high-risk period for weight gain. Brush your teeth after dinner to mentally signal to yourself that your eating has finished for the day.

Improve the quality of sleep by darkening the room, avoiding screen time too close to bedtime, and keeping the bedroom cooler.

> **Tip #22:** Increase both duration and quality of sleep.

INCRETINS, PEPTIDE YY, AND CHOLECYSTOKININ: THE SATIETY HORMONES

THERE'S A POPULAR BELIEF that humans are eating machines, designed, like The Blob from that old horror movie, to eat everything in front of us. Now that food is so easily available, goes this belief, we eat too much and therefore become obese. This overeating can't be helped. It's the price of living in the modern world. If you don't think too hard about it, this idea seems plausible. Under thoughtful scrutiny, its truthful façade melts like a Popsicle on a hot summer's day.

We obviously don't just eat everything we see. We stop eating when we are full. The human body has multiple powerful overlapping satiety mechanisms that tell us to stop eating. Think about a time you've eaten way, way too much food at an all-you-can-eat buffet. Even as you're stuffed to the gills, your friend says: "Hey, just eat these two pork chops, or we'll get charged for them." The very thought nauseates you. Yet these are the very same pork chops that you hungrily ate just minutes ago.

Eating one hamburger is delicious. Eating twenty hamburgers is near impossible for most people. Why? Because when you've had enough to eat, your body secretes powerful satiety hormones—incretins, peptide YY, and cholecystokinin—that strongly discourage you from eating any more. These hormones are the reason we stop eating.

The incretins: GLP-1 and GIP

The incretin hormones, including glucagon-like peptide 1 (GLP-1) and glucose-dependent insulinotropic polypeptide (GIP), are released by intestinal cells and signal us to stop eating. More recently, a synthetic incretin similar to GLP-1 has been developed from the venom of the Gila monster, a small poisonous lizard native to the American southwest. This drug, called semaglutide, also known as Ozempic, has become a blockbuster weight-loss medication that could increase the effect of GLP-1 to very high levels.

Incretins lead to weight loss through three main mechanisms:

1. Slowed gastric emptying
2. Increased satiety
3. Nausea and vomiting

First, the incretins reduce how quickly the stomach empties, keeping the baroreceptors stretched longer, which makes us feel full for longer.[14,15] The delayed nutrient absorption flattens the rise in blood glucose (and insulin) after meals. Slower absorption of nutrients leads to less glucose and fewer insulin spikes. Less insulin means less fat storage. Second, the incretins increase satiety by activating neurons in the brain's appetite center in the hypothalamus, particularly the sub-fornical organ. The neurons signal fullness and reduce the amount we eat. Third, the incretins affect the area postrema, which makes you feel nauseated, sometimes to the point of vomiting. Nausea can't really be considered a side effect, since a rather stunning 89.7 percent of participants taking Ozempic experienced it. It's truly how this drug works.

Together, these three mechanisms powerfully reduce our desire to eat. With Ozempic, you lose your appetite, feel a bit nauseated, and when/if you eat, you stay full longer. According to a 2023 Morgan Stanley research survey, people taking Ozempic ate about 1000 fewer calories per day.[16] They ate fewer meals and snacks, ate out less, and chose healthier foods—more fruits, vegetables, fish, and chicken—and fewer confections, sugary drinks, cookies, alcohol, and salty snacks (potato chips). Ozempic lowers insulin levels by almost 50 percent because people are eating so much less food.[17]

What can we learn from the success of Ozempic? **Successful long-term weight loss is NOT about controlling calories but about controlling hunger and satiety.** Ozempic does not reduce calories directly. Bariatric surgery physically restricts calories, but it is relatively ineffective for lasting weight loss. Ozempic reduces hunger, which reduces eating behavior, which reduces calories. This is a crucial distinction. If you simply eat fewer calories, your hunger may increase and compel you to eat more calories. Eating fewer calories won't lead to long-term weight loss. Ozempic works at the root cause; it reduces the hunger. A newer drug called tirzepatide, also known as Mounjaro, stimulates both the GLP-1 and GIP hormones and has shown even better weight-loss effects.

Peptide YY and cholecystokinin

Peptide YY (PYY) and cholecystokinin (CCK) are both gut hormones that regulate digestion and appetite. When we eat proteins and fats, intestinal cells release peptide YY and cholecystokinin, which slows stomach emptying and reduces appetite through its effects on the brain (nucleus tractus solitarius and arcuate nucleus of the hypothalamus).[18]

ADRENALINE AND NORADRENALINE:
THE SYMPATHETIC NERVOUS SYSTEM

MANY OF THE body's automatic functions, like your heartbeat or breathing, are regulated by the autonomic nervous system. The autonomic nervous system has two main divisions, the parasympathetic nervous system (PNS) and the sympathetic nervous system (SNS). These systems are complementary: the PNS prepares the body for rest, digestion, and maintenance (the "rest-and-digest" response) and the sympathetic nervous system (SNS) prepares the body for action (the "fight-or-flight" response).

The SNS increases our chances of survival when confronted by a lion, for example. The SNS releases hormones such as adrenaline and noradrenaline that prepare the body either to fight or to run fast. Activating the SNS increases the body's awareness, arousal, and available energy (glucose) as your heart beats faster, you breathe more quickly, and you prepare for action. When the SNS is activated, you expend more energy and burn fat (lipolysis) to provide that energy. The SNS also powerfully suppresses your appetite and hunger.

When you're in danger—suddenly confronted by a lion or a gang of criminals—do you suddenly think, "Oh, I'm a bit peckish"? Do you ever feel hungry while playing an intense game of basketball or hockey? No! Blood is diverted away from your body's hunger and digestion response to focus on supplying the muscles with energy. Your sympathetic tone, the activity level of the sympathetic nerves, is high.

Certain drugs activate the SNS to cause weight loss. The most common example is nicotine. While smoking nicotine is super unhealthy, it does cause weight loss. People who smoke are thinner than people who have never smoked. Studies show that when smokers quit, their weight rises over ten years to closely mirror the weight of non-smokers (Figure 4.3[19]).[20] The difference is not the calories; it is the reduced level of stimulation of the hormones—sympathetic tone—that is affecting the body fat thermostat.

Figure 4.3. Average changes in body mass index over ten years for smokers, former smokers, and non-smokers

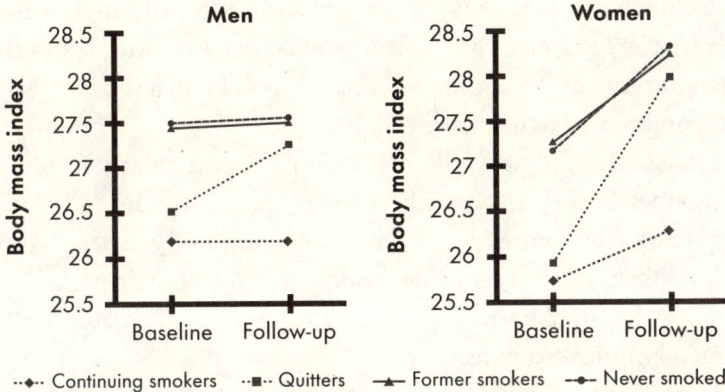

··◆·· Continuing smokers   ··■·· Quitters   ▬▲▬ Former smokers   ▬●▬ Never smoked

In the 1990s, the notorious weight-loss drug fen-phen (fenfluramine + phentermine, both of which activate the SNS) was widely prescribed because it produced an average weight loss of 15 to 18 percent of initial weight.[21] That kind of weight loss is on par with the modern "miracle" drug Ozempic. Over four years, some patients kept an average of 30 pounds (14 kg) of weight off. Like Ozempic, fen-phen does not restrict calories; it reduces hunger. Phentermine releases norepinephrine, and fenfluramine releases serotonin, which increase sympathetic tone and therefore lower the body fat thermostat so that the body maintains a lower weight. Despite its effectiveness as a weight-loss drug, however, fen-phen was eventually withdrawn from the market in 1997 because it caused severe heart problems.[22]

Another drug that suppresses appetite is methamphetamine (street name "speed") and its more recent form crystal meth, an illegal and highly addictive stimulant. It belongs to a class of drugs called anorexiants, which suppress appetite by activating the SNS. When people stop taking methamphetamine (or crystal meth), they rapidly regain weight. The difference is not willpower; the difference is the hunger. Activating

73

the SNS lowers the body fat thermostat. When the SNS is no longer actively stimulated, the body fat thermostat rises.

The opposite effect happens with drugs that block SNS. Beta blockers, commonly used for heart disease, block the SNS and are associated with an average weight gain of 2.6 pounds (1.2 kg).[23] Antidepressants, which increase blood serotonin levels, are well known to cause weight gain, sometimes large amounts.[24]

Exercise does temporarily boost the SNS, particularly in competitive games, and this effect is known as "exercise-induced anorexia." This effect is temporary but useful. For example, if you are planning to skip lunch, you can schedule a game of tennis to help get over the hunger that will likely occur. Competitive exercise is a natural, albeit temporary, hunger suppressant.

> **Tip #23:** Use moderate exercise to temporarily control hunger.

TESTOSTERONE, ESTROGEN, PROGESTERONE: THE SEX HORMONES

PRIOR TO PUBERTY, boys and girls have roughly the same body fat percentage. After puberty, girls gain about 50 percent more fat than boys, distributed mostly in the hips and thighs in preparation for childbearing. Boys gain more muscle, which becomes obvious in sports. The difference does not arise due to calories or willpower, but from the difference in sex hormones.

During puberty, girls produce more estrogen and boys produce more testosterone. Estrogen diverts more calories toward storage as body fat, especially in the breasts, hips, and thighs. Testosterone diverts calories into muscle growth. Usually that means boys must eat more (and teenage boys eat a *lot*). It's not exercise, willpower, or calories that matter. The difference is the hormones that instruct the body what to do with those calories.

Men with the higher levels of testosterone have more muscle and less fat.[25] During androgen deprivation therapy for prostate cancer, testosterone levels are pushed to very low levels. This low testosterone slows down the cancer growth but also causes men to gain 11 percent more body fat and lose 3.8 percent of lean mass.[26]

How the menstrual cycle affects appetite and weight gain

Changes in hormones during the menstrual cycle also affect eating behavior. Estrogen slowly rises at the beginning of the cycle and peaks midway through ovulation. Estrogen is known to decrease appetite, and women, on average, eat less during the first part of their menstrual cycle. After ovulation, progesterone rises, which stimulates hunger, and women generally eat more. Megestrol, a synthetic form of progesterone, is sometimes given to cancer patients to stimulate their appetite which results in weight gain. How many calories we eat depends on the hormonal instructions the body receives. The problem is the hunger, not the calories.

Changes in estrogen levels also influence weight gain in perimenopausal and menopausal women. Women typically gain 2.25 kg (5 pounds) of weight during the perimenopausal period.[27] As estrogen goes down, weight is redistributed back from the fat under the skin around the hips and thighs and breasts to the visceral fat, particularly around the abdomen. Estrogen reduces appetite, so the lower estrogen during menopause increases appetite. Women eat more, and so tend to gain weight. Perimenopausal weight gain is not about "eating too many calories" or having "too little willpower" but has everything to do with the lower estrogen levels.

We cannot always manipulate the sex hormones for weight loss, but knowing about these changes bolsters the overwhelming evidence that weight gain is not as simplistic as Calories In, Calories Out. However, hormone replacement therapy for menopausal women can be controversial, and the role of testosterone replacement in older men is yet to be defined.

75

THYROID HORMONES

THE THYROID HORMONES influence the body's metabolic rate, regulating the speed of digestion and how much energy (calories) you burn. An overactive thyroid (hyperthyroidism) causes your metabolic rate to increase, with symptoms such as sweating, nervousness, tremor, irritability, and weight loss. An underactive thyroid (hypothyroidism) reduces your metabolic rate and can causes symptoms like fatigue, constipation, cold intolerance, and weight gain.

We cannot directly influence our thyroid function by the foods we eat or by manipulating thyroid hormones, but these hormones are involved with weight gain and loss nevertheless.

HYPOGLYCEMIC HUNGER

HYPOGLYCEMIA IS A condition of low blood sugars, often caused by an imbalance of insulin and glucose, and it causes shaking, sweating, and profound hunger. Blood glucose levels almost always stay in the normal range for most people, except in two specific situations:

1. You are taking medications to lower blood glucose.
2. You experience reactive hypoglycemia.

If you are taking medications to regulate blood glucose, and you don't manage them properly, blood glucose can fall too low and you experience hypoglycemia.

After a sudden spike in glucose and insulin, followed by an equally violent drop, some people will experience a reactive hypoglycemia that takes their blood glucose below normal. This type of hypoglycemia most commonly happens when we eat highly refined carbohydrates. In a classic 1977 scientific experiment, apple juice, but not whole apples or applesauce, caused hypoglycemia (Figure 4.4[28]).[29]

Figure 4.4. Blood glucose levels rise more and drop lower after drinking apple juice compared with less processed foods

**Effects of food processing
on plasma glucose levels**

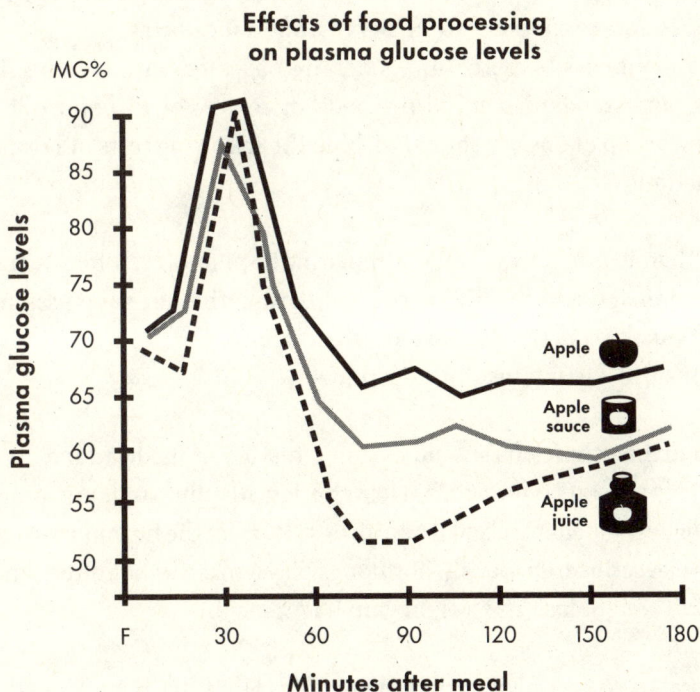

Similarly, if you eat two slices of white bread and jam with orange juice in the morning, you'll find yourself famished by 10:30 a.m. and looking for a low-fat muffin to soothe your hunger pangs. Your blood glucose rocketed higher because you ate highly refined carbohydrates with nothing else (naked carbs), and then crashed, causing hypoglycemia.

The best way to avoid hypoglycemic hunger is to avoid eating rapidly digestible starches. Instead, choose low Glycemic Index starches with plenty of fiber. Alternatively, eating two eggs with bacon in the morning will keep you full at least until noon.

Simply not eating (fasting) does not generally cause hypoglycemia. The human body stores food energy (calories) in two forms: glucose and triglycerides (body fat). If you don't eat for a while, you'll deplete your stored glucose first and then simply switch to using body fat for energy.

The bottom line is that homeostatic hunger is governed by hormones and, to a lesser extent, nerves, but not calories.

Weight-loss "experts" are generally obsessed with calories. However, any standard medical textbook or review[30] will point out that any workup of obesity should include the following tests of hormonal function:

- Thyroid function: thyroid-stimulating hormone (TSH), free T3, free T4
- Adrenal function: urinary cortisol, dexamethasone suppression test
- Gonadal function: testosterone, estrogen
- Insulin: fasting insulin, C-peptide

Further, clinicians should ask for a history of medications, such as antidepressants, steroids, antipsychotics, insulin, smoking, amphetamines, and beta blockers. These drugs all affect the hormonal systems we've described. Obviously, hormones play a massive but often ignored role in weight loss and weight gain (Figure 4.5).

Figure 4.5. A constellation of hormones affect body fat, but calories do not

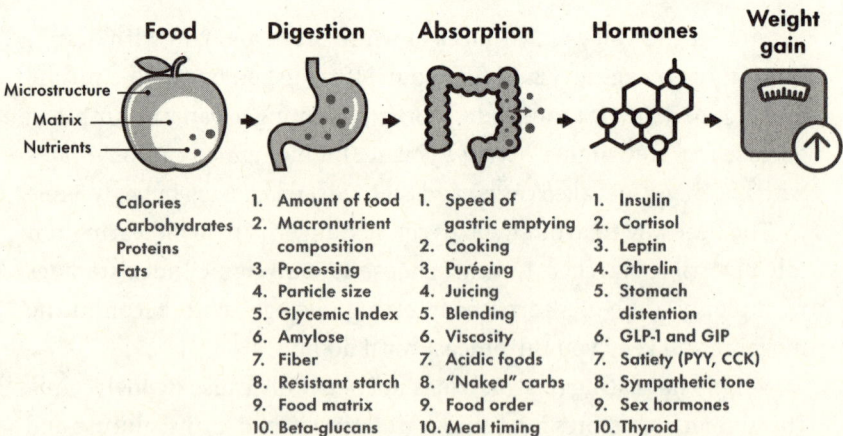

Food	Digestion	Absorption	Hormones	Weight gain
Microstructure — Matrix — Nutrients —				
Calories	1. Amount of food	1. Speed of gastric emptying	1. Insulin	
Carbohydrates	2. Macronutrient composition	2. Cooking	2. Cortisol	
Proteins	3. Processing	3. Puréeing	3. Leptin	
Fats	4. Particle size	4. Juicing	4. Ghrelin	
	5. Glycemic Index	5. Blending	5. Stomach distention	
	6. Amylose	6. Viscosity	6. GLP-1 and GIP	
	7. Fiber	7. Acidic foods	7. Satiety (PYY, CCK)	
	8. Resistant starch	8. "Naked" carbs	8. Sympathetic tone	
	9. Food matrix	9. Food order	9. Sex hormones	
	10. Beta-glucans	10. Meal timing	10. Thyroid	

One factor is highly notable for its absence: calories. Calories are physiologically and medically meaningless. The problem was never the calories. That's why calorie restriction never worked. The human body doesn't care about calories. The human body doesn't count calories. The hormones are the key.

Over the years, many proposed treatments for obesity have reduced calories, often by physically restricting the number of calories that could enter the body. In the 1970s and 1980s, wiring the jaw shut was a popular weight-loss solution.[31] It caused severe physical and emotional distress, dental problems, and gum disease, but didn't really work. People quickly regained all their lost weight when their jaws were opened. The same experience took place with bariatric surgery several decades later. Bulimia is also a desperate attempt at calorie control. Vomiting after meals reduces calories in the body, but it does not lead to long-term weight loss.

So why don't these weight-loss methods work? Because all these treatments are based on the underlying, incorrect premise that reducing calories is the most important thing for weight loss.

On the other hand, there are drugs that will reliably cause weight loss, including nicotine, speed, crystal meth, Ozempic (semaglutide), Mounjaro (tirzepatide), and fen-phen. None of these effective drugs target calories. They all affect the hormones that drive the body fat thermostat. There are also some medications that reliably cause weight gain: insulin, cortisol, beta blockers, antidepressants. What do they all have in common? Hormones.

After asking and answering the three "whys" of weight loss, the conclusion is that obesity is a hormonal, not a caloric, imbalance. Successful treatment for obesity depends upon fixing this root cause. Manage the hunger, not the calories.

| 5 |

MANAGING HUNGER,
NOT CALORIES

H AVE YOU EVER eaten a loaf of garlic bread, a bowl of pasta, and a tub of pistachio gelato and still felt hungry? Have you ever finished dinner and then secretly eaten a bag of potato chips before bed? You're not alone. I hear these stories every day. Your mind tells you that you should be full, but your stomach still complains that it's empty. You feel helpless and out of control, bingeing on foods you know you should be avoiding.

The opposite happens as well. Some people eat half a sandwich or a small salad at lunchtime and then feel completely stuffed. They're not trying to be modest. They won't eat more because it is uncomfortable for them to do so. It's not willpower; it's physiology.

What you eat determines *how much* you eat. If you eat a lot of foods that fill you up, you can't eat any more. There are strong satiety hormones that stop you. If you eat foods that don't fill you up, you'll eat more and more often. There are even foods that make you hungrier. This difference can be surprisingly significant: studies have found up to a seven-fold difference in the satiating effect of different foods.[1]

Different foods with the same calories produce different levels of satiety. Some foods make you full and others don't, for the simple reason that they affect the neurohormonal satiety mechanisms completely differently. We eat because we are hungry. We stop eating when we are full. This is obvious, and we all know this fact, of course. Drinking 500 calories of soda pop does not reduce hunger, whereas eating a 500-calorie hamburger patty does. So why pretend that all calories are the same? A calorie is not a calorie.

Eating more satiating foods is the key to adjusting the body fat thermostat down to a healthy weight, and keeping it there so that weight does not creep up. The question is, what should you eat and drink to feel more full? Unfortunately, no easy answer exists, but hey, that's life. You can either reach for the simple, but incorrect, answer or strive to understand the complex but correct one. Here are a few specifics to keep in mind.

EAT NATURAL FATS AND PROTEIN

WE'VE DISCUSSED CARBOHYDRATES at length, so let's consider the other two macronutrients—dietary fat and protein. For a further discussion, see *The Obesity Code*.

Natural dietary fat is good

Sir William Osler (1849–1919) is often called the Father of Modern Medicine. In his classic 1892 textbook, *The Principles and Practice of Medicine*, his recommended treatment for obesity was a diet of 65 percent fat, 32 percent protein, and 3 percent carbohydrates.[2] He believed that eating enough fat increased satiety and was therefore crucial in the treatment of obesity. Dr. Osler was far ahead of his time, and quite correct. Eating fat releases the satiety hormones peptide YY, cholecystokinin, and incretins.

Olive oil, for example, strongly stimulates the incretin hormones GLP-1[3] and GIP.[4] A Mediterranean diet rich in olive oil reduces insulin and doubles GLP-1 compared to a carbohydrate-rich diet, despite identical calories.[5] A low-carbohydrate, high healthy fat diet releases about 50 percent more peptide YY compared to a high-carb, low-fat diet.[6]

81

Despite clear evidence that natural fat is *good* for our health, many people have come to believe otherwise. Why? Since 1961, the American Heart Association has been recommending that we eat less dietary fat and saturated fat.[7] Saturated fat, which occurs naturally as coconut oil, butter, and animal fats, was demonized. Instead, ostensibly to reduce heart disease, Americans were encouraged to switch to margarines made with the then-newfangled hydrogenated vegetable oils, also known as trans fats.

Then the U.S. government's 1977 dietary guidelines urged Americans to eat less fat and more refined carbohydrates, in the mistaken belief that it would eradicate heart disease. More bread. More rice. More potatoes. Next, in the early 1990s, the U.S. Department of Agriculture introduced the food pyramid, a visual guide to the recommended daily servings from various food groups. The pyramid advised us to eat six to eleven portions daily from the Bread, Cereal, Rice & Pasta Group. Americans didn't *choose* to eat more refined carbs. They were *told* to eat more refined carbs. And like trusting calves to the slaughter, Americans listened.

No actual scientific evidence at the time supported the claim that we should eat less fat,[8] and no subsequent studies supported this contention either. Some people had pointed out, as obesity rates rose in the U.S. in the 1980s, the so-called French paradox. How was it, they wondered, that people in decadent France could enjoy a diet filled with natural fats like butter and cream and also enjoy a rate of heart disease and obesity far lower than virtuous, low-fat America? There was no paradox. It was simple. Eating natural fat doesn't cause heart disease and eating less fat doesn't reduce heart disease. Eating natural fat doesn't cause obesity and eating less doesn't reduce obesity.

What does matter is that the fats be naturally occurring—like the fats in coconut oil, chia seeds, avocados, butter, and animal fats—rather than industrial. Some call them "healthy" fats, but that term lacks specificity. Industrial seed oils, such as cottonseed, sunflower, and soy, are cheap to produce but they often involve chemical processing. For example, the oils are extracted from the seeds using petroleum-based hexane solvents, then the oils are refined by bleaching, deodorizing, and degumming. Some of these fats are then hydrogenated or partially hydrogenated to make them solid at room temperature. Adding hydrogen to liquid fat changes its chemical composition, turning it into a trans fatty acid (trans fat). Not good.

By the 1990s, new studies discovered that for every 2 percent increase in trans fats consumption, the risk of heart disease increased by a staggering 23 percent. The trans fats were causing an estimated 76,000 to 228,000 excess heart attacks. Every year![9] The very "heart-healthy" foods the "experts" insisted we eat were *causing*, not preventing, heart disease. The irony, the irony. By November 2013, the U.S. Food and Drug Administration removed partially hydrogenated oils from the list of human foods "generally recognized as safe." Yes, the "experts" had been telling us to eat poison *for decades*.

The results of the huge eighteen-country Prospective Urban Rural Epidemiology (PURE) study, which looked at the relationship between macronutrients and cardiovascular disease, were released in 2017.[10] They further confirmed that eating a low-fat diet was associated with more, not less, heart disease.

Nutritional orthodoxy changes every few years, but it's hard to go wrong with eating natural fats that have been part of the human diet since antiquity. Again, these natural fats include animal fats, butter, dairy fats, fatty fish (like mackerel and salmon), walnuts, almonds, avocados, and coconut oil. But don't eat more fat than necessary, past the point of satiety. Dietary fat is absorbed into the lymphatic system, which empties into the bloodstream and is then taken up by the fat cells (adipocytes). Thus, any fat you eat must still be burned off.

One particularly nasty trap are foods labeled "low fat" or "fat free." They're usually highly processed and loaded with sugars or other additives. In order to use less fat, food companies usually use chemicals like texturizers or emulsifiers to get the right mouthfeel and then sugar to distract you. Eating the natural, full-fat version is almost always a better choice.

> **Tip #24:** Don't fear natural fats, but don't eat more
> than necessary. Avoid foods labeled "low fat" or "fat free."

Natural dietary protein is also good—in moderation

Dietary protein increases the satiety hormones more than the other macronutrients.[11] It also increases metabolism (diet-induced thermogenesis). Harvard researcher Dr. Frank Hu wrote: "There is convincing evidence that a higher protein intake increases thermogenesis and satiety compared to diets of lower protein content. The weight of evidence also suggests that high protein meals lead to a reduced subsequent energy intake."[12] In other words, eating protein makes you feel more full, increases metabolism,[13] and decreases the amount you want to eat later.

This effect is particularly noticeable at morning breakfast and when eating branched-chain amino acids, such as the ones found in dairy. Research shows that a high-protein (30%) diet stimulates more GLP-1 and keeps people fuller for longer compared to an equal-calorie lower-protein diet.[14] So eating breakfast in the morning and including protein—such as eggs, Greek yogurt, or meat—is a more effective way to keep you full for the day than eating toast or sugary cereals. To feel more full, choose animal over vegetable proteins.[15]

In the same way that many people have heard eating dietary fat is bad, they have also heard that eating more protein is good. The Recommended Daily Allowance, the official recommendation for good health, for protein is 0.8 g/kg of body weight per day. The average American eats between 1.2 and 1.4 g/kg/day, or nearly double the recommended amount. Put another way, we need roughly 32 to 46 grams of dietary protein every day for body maintenance, and the average American eats 65 to 100+ grams.[16] When we digest that protein, our bodies break it down into amino acids. However, we can't store amino acids, and so excess protein must be changed into glucose by the liver. An estimated 50 to 70 percent of the protein the average American eats is therefore turned into glucose. Thus, eating excessive protein is not much better than eating excessive glucose.[17,18]

Americans are not alone in eating too much protein. In 2021, China surpassed the U.S. for number of grams of protein eaten per person per day (per capita), reaching 124.61 grams. Roughly two-thirds of the protein eaten in China is plant based, compared to the U.S.'s one-third, but plant-based protein doesn't seem to protect against weight gain. China now also faces a worsening obesity epidemic.[19]

Eating a very high protein, low-fat, low-carbohydrate diet is difficult to stick with, because it just doesn't taste very good. The fat that accompanies meat protein significantly improves its flavor and texture, which is why the fattiest cuts of beef (like USDA AAA or Prime) are the most prized and expensive. Skin-on chicken is tastier than chicken breast. For flavor, fatty tuna is far preferred over lean tuna. Eggs, cottage cheese, and Greek yogurt are all good options. The highest-protein vegetable sources include tofu, lentils, dried beans, spelt, and spirulina.

> **Tip #25:** Prioritize a moderate amount of protein for its neurohormonal satiety effects (GLP-1, PYY, and CCK).

Protein powders are best avoided

Protein powders promise protein without much carbohydrate or fat. Unfortunately, eating ultra-processed protein powder is not the same as eating naturally high-protein foods.

Multiple studies have concluded that protein powders, such as whey or soy protein, provide satiety but little weight loss.[20] Protein powders increase GLP-1 and peptide YY, but do not reduce how much people eat, although the reasons remain unclear.[21] Protein supplements also don't help weight loss after bariatric surgery, and neither do they seem to improve muscle mass significantly.[22] And a meta-analysis similarly showed a lack of benefit for weight loss in post-menopausal women.[23]

85

As with carbohydrates, the food matrix (the physical structure of the food) plays an important role in satiety for proteins. Protein powders are often made by processing cheap plant or animal products to isolate the protein, which means removing naturally occurring carbs, fats, fiber, and other beneficial nutrients and then sometimes adding sweeteners or other additives. So protein powders are very different from high-protein foods. My best advice is to avoid protein powders and eat "whole" natural proteins, recognizing that there is a limit to how much you can realistically eat, both from a cost perspective as well as a palatability one.

> **Tip #26:** Eat naturally protein-rich foods, not ultra-processed protein powders.

ADD BITTER FOODS TO YOUR DIET

BITTERNESS IN FOOD is thought to be a natural warning against potential toxins. However, many bitter foods are well liked, including dark chocolate, coffee and green tea (see more about these drinks below), kale, arugula, watercress, eggplant, Brussels sprouts, and citrus peel. Bitter compounds increase cholecystokinin and GLP-1, reduce ghrelin, and slow the rate at which the stomach empties. All these actions reduce appetite and food cravings and increase satiety.[24] Some research has shown that curcumin, the active ingredient in turmeric, directly stimulates GLP-1[25] up to 30 percent[26] and can help with modest weight loss.[27]

Bitter foods are difficult to overindulge because the bitterness builds up. For example, I love the flavor of eggplant and arugula, but I can't keep eating them forever as I could with ice cream, because the bitterness eventually becomes unpleasant. This effect is likely part of the reason why eating more bitter foods helps overall health. Some people are more sensitive than others to the chemical compounds called glucosinolates that create the bitter taste in foods. Our sensitivity generally decreases as we age, which is why adults often enjoy bitter foods that kids spit out, so enjoy these foods as your taste and your tolerance allow.

> **Tip #27:** Eat more bitter foods, including turmeric.

DRINK MORE TEA

TEA IS ONE of the world's most popular beverages, having spread along trade routes from China to Europe and England, and then out to colonial outposts around the world. Legend claims that the original cup of tea was an accident discovered when the first Yan Emperor, Shen Nong, was boiling water in a pot and some leaves fell in. This slightly bitter drink made him think quicker and see clearer, and tea drinking subsequently went "viral" (or at least the equivalent 5000 years ago).

The Chinese called this drink "tu," meaning bitter, and similar words have carried over to many languages, from the English "tea" to the Maori "tii." In the mid seventh century, a pen stroke was removed from the Chinese word to become "cha," and this word traveled from the dialects of the landlocked regions in China with merchants who plied the Silk Roads. It has become the Swahili "chai" and Russian "chay." Virtually everywhere in the world, in fact, tea is known by a variation of "tu" or "cha." In addition to its calming effect, tea boosts metabolism and can fill your stomach so you feel more full.

Prefer green tea, and also oolong and black teas

Green tea is made from freshly harvested leaves of the *Camellia sinensis* plant that are immediately steamed, rolled, and dried. This tea has a high concentration of polyphenols and powerful antioxidants called catechins, 50 to 80 percent of which is epigallocatechin-3-gallate. The green tea leaves can be partially fermented to become oolong tea or further fermented to become black tea. Fermentation changes the polyphenols and catechins to theaflavins, which may have their own beneficial effects.

Many studies show that drinking green tea helps weight loss[28,29] through several mechanisms:

1. Increases metabolic rate and fat oxidation (increased sympathetic tone)
2. Decreases hunger/appetite (decreased ghrelin)
3. Blocks glucose absorption

The catechins in green tea block the enzyme called catechol-O-methyltransferase (COMT), which normally deactivates adrenaline and noradrenaline, the hormones of the sympathetic nervous system that rev up metabolism. So blocking COMT allows noradrenaline levels to stay higher. This effect works together with the caffeine in green tea to increase metabolic rate by 4 to 5 percent[30,31,32] and reduce hunger. Similarly, the theaflavins in oolong tea are shown to raise energy expenditure by 2.9 percent.[33] Some studies suggest that this metabolic boost may be larger for Asians who, genetically, have higher COMT activity.[34,35]

In addition to the hunger-reducing effect of activating the sympathetic nervous system, green tea also lowers ghrelin.[36] The combined effect of increasing metabolism and decreasing the hunger-stimulating hormone leads the body to burn off more energy, which helps to lower weight and the body fat thermostat.

Finally, to reduce glucose absorption, catechins inhibit the enzymes amylase and glucosidase. This effect can lower glucose absorption by up to 25 percent. Both green and black teas block carbohydrate absorption, which is exactly what we want for weight loss and type 2 diabetes.[37]

The weight-loss benefits of tea are not huge, but the risks are virtually non-existent. Why *wouldn't* you drink more tea? I can't think of a single reason. Battles are always won on the margin, and small benefits multiplied over many years can add up. Try to drink three or more cups of tea per day. When at home, I keep some tea leaves in my strainer all day long and simply add hot water every time I want to drink something. In the summer, I prefer my tea cold. I make a big pot of green tea, add some strawberries to infuse flavor, and keep it in the fridge.

Herbal teas are great drinks, but they are not true teas since they don't contain the leaf of the tea plant. While they may still have significant benefits, they have been less studied than green or black teas.

Drink cold-brewed tea as well as hot

Although the cold-brew process is more familiar for coffee drinkers, you can use it with tea to extract more of the beneficial catechins. Cold-brewing coffee means allowing the coarsely ground beans to steep in cold water for hours or even days, to gently release the compounds which results in a smoother-tasting, less acidic coffee.

Similarly, cold-brewing tea extracts more fully the delicate polyphenols and catechins responsible for much of the metabolic benefits. Simply steep green tea in room temperature water for six hours to draw more of the catechins out. Cold-brewing green tea extracts two to three times the amount of catechins compared to hot water brewing. And this "whole foods" method of cold brewing preserves all the natural elements of the tea in balance compared with industrially processed green tea extracts.

> **Tip #28:** Drink lots of green, oolong, and black tea.

DRINK MORE COFFEE

COFFEE CONTAINS MORE of the stimulant caffeine than tea does, which increases fat oxidation and metabolism by up to 10 percent.[38] Each additional cup of coffee is associated with weight loss of 0.12 kg (0.26 pounds), although adding sugar or flavored syrups lessens this benefit.[39] Coffee has many antioxidants and contains chlorogenic acid, which inhibits the enzymes alpha-glucosidase and glucose-6-phosphatase, so carbohydrates are absorbed more slowly.[40]

The caffeine in coffee is usually released over fifteen to forty-five minutes. That release is much faster than tea, which releases its caffeine over several hours. The rapid absorption and peak may disrupt sleep, so you may want to drink coffee earlier in the day.

Like tea, coffee can be cold brewed for a smoother drink and served cold in the summer. Drinking more coffee (and tea) also reduces the tendency to drink sodas, juices, or other sugary beverages. Green tea and coffee are the best beverages of all for controlling hunger.

Tip #29: Drink more coffee.

DRINK SPARKLING WATER MINDFULLY

BRING ON THE BUBBLES! Drinking carbonated or sparkling water, like San Pellegrino or Perrier, has been popular in Europe for many years, and the trend seems to have taken off in North America too. Does drinking sparkling water help with weight loss?

This is a difficult question to answer, since few scientific studies currently exist. A small study in 2017 involving only twenty participants noted that carbonated water, even unflavored, increased ghrelin release. This finding suggests that sparkling water could stimulate appetite, which is not good for weight loss.[41] However, this small study hasn't been replicated, so the best advice I can give is to simply try to assess the effects of drinking sparkling water on your own hunger. If drinking carbonated water doesn't seem to increase your hunger, then continue.

Avoid diet sodas

For decades, the diet food industry has promised that you can enjoy sodas and other sweet foods without gaining weight. First, there was saccharin. In the 1980s, aspartame and phenylalanine were introduced, followed by sucralose in 1998, then stevia and monk fruit extracts in the 2000s. Replacing sugar with low-calorie sweeteners (LCS) seems like such a good idea for weight loss. But it has failed. Miserably.

In the Nurses' Health Study, a large, long-term prospective study, people taking the most LCS gained 54 percent more weight than those taking the least.[42] In the San Antonio Heart Study, weight gain was 78 percent higher.[43] When all randomized controlled trials were reviewed, scientists concluded that "sweetener had no significant effect on BMI."[44] Yes, you could have a drink with zero calories, but no, it didn't help you lose weight. Why? Because the problem has never been the calories. The problem is the hunger, and taking more LCS makes you hungrier.

Both regular soda and diet soda increase ghrelin three- to fourfold compared to plain water.[45] However, the lack of calories in the diet soda leaves people unfulfilled and seeking those calories. A 2025 study using brain scans explained further that, "unlike sugar, sucralose did not increase blood levels of certain hormones that create a feeling of fullness. The findings show how sucralose confuses the brain by providing a sweet taste without the expected caloric energy."[46] Sucralose "increased hunger and activity in the hypothalamus," the brain structure critical for hunger. Sugar increases GLP-1 and induces satiety, but sucralose does not.

Essentially, the LCS messes up your brain, tricking it into thinking that calories are coming. When they don't, you are left hungrier and look for more food to compensate. That's why diet drinks and foods never cause weight loss. Let's use some common sense. Suppose you buy a case of diet soda to replace your regular soda. Twenty-four cans of regular soda totals about 4800 calories. Have you ever noticed that you've lost 1.5 pounds (0.68 kg) of fat for each case of diet soda you've drunk? Doubtful. In 2023, the World Health Organization unequivocally advised against using "non-sugar sweeteners for weight control."[47] Why? Because they don't help you lose weight. People who drink diet compared to regular soda eat roughly the same total number of calories per day, despite the zero calories of the diet soda.[48]

91

Tip #30: Avoid "diet" sodas and "sugar-free" foods.

HOW TO EAT FOR SATIETY
AND AVOID HOMEOSTATIC HUNGER

EATING FOR SATIETY is not about restricting calories or eating specially designed foods; it's about making food choices that enhance your body's own processes for regulating hunger and fullness. When we eat foods that make us feel full and trigger the body's own satiety hormones, we naturally stop eating. No calorie counting, no willpower, no drama required. Intuitively, we know this. Simple, natural, whole foods produce the greatest satiety. When we eat fish, steak, fruits, boiled potatoes, dried beans, lentils, cheese, or eggs, we feel full.[49]

When you're trying to lose weight or maintain it, pick foods that are

1. bulky—high volume (take up space) and low energy density (full of fiber and water),
2. more time-consuming to chew and swallow,
3. natural, without additives,
4. higher in protein,
5. higher in fiber,
6. lower in sugar,
7. lower on the Glycemic Index, and
8. heavy (create a feeling of weight in the stomach).

The problem? We live in a white bread world. In other words, we want foods that are cheap, convenient, have a long shelf life, and are easy to chew and swallow. These foods—breakfast cereals, pasta, pizza, not to mention potato chips, cookies, and chocolate bars—stimulate insulin a lot and satiety only a little. That's a lethal combination for weight gain. The problem is that the modern Western diet prioritizes price and convenience, not health.

Standard nutrition labels provide information about calories, but they don't provide information about satiety or about the three factors that most contribute to weight gain: energy density, eating rate, and hyper-palatability.[50] Energy-dense foods provide quick fuel for the body. Think, for example, chocolate bars or high-sugar energy bars. Eating rate is the speed at which you consume foods. In our fast-paced world, we wolf down snacks between one meeting and the next or mindlessly devour our meal on the way out the door. The faster we eat foods, the faster they reach the stomach. And hyper-palatable foods are designed to smell good, feel good, and taste good, even if it means adding chemicals—artificial colors and artificial flavors—to achieve those results.

As we'll see in the next part of the book, even if we know what we *should* be eating, actually doing that can be much harder. Food manufacturers specifically engineer foods for quick energy, quick eating, and maximum flavor, and they make those foods cheap and easy to find. The problem is that these ultra-processed foods are delicious but they don't make us feel full. The result? We keep eating and eating and eating...for pleasure and for comfort.

HARRY

Harry was a forty-five-year-old man who had done many diets. He'd previously lost weight by following a keto diet or through intermittent fasting, but he could never keep the weight off long term.

When he came to see me, Harry weighed 225 pounds (102 kg). His goal was to reach and maintain a healthy weight for him, which meant about 180 pounds (82 kg).

He started with twenty-two-hour fasts three times a week and was gradually able to extend each of those fasts to forty hours. After three months, he had lost 3.5 inches (9 cm) from around his waist, had more energy, and was no longer snoring, which his wife appreciated! More importantly, he'd spent time learning how eating carbs first in a meal caused him to overeat and experience insulin spikes.

By eating carbs after other foods and combining them with vinegar, he'd learned to slow the speed at which his body digested and absorbed those carbs, reducing insulin spikes and lowering his body fat thermostat. This time, he also surrounded himself with supportive friends and lifestyle coaches. Addressing the root causes of his weight gain, adopting new habits, and creating a support network gave Harry confidence that he could not only reach a healthy weight but also maintain it.

CATHY

Cathy was in her fifties when she joined The Fasting Method to lose weight. She had been dieting since her teens and was diagnosed with type 2 diabetes in her early thirties. To manage the diabetes, she'd been prescribed metformin, two types of insulin, and eventually a GLP-1 medication. Although Cathy had lost some weight while taking the GLP-1 drug, none of the drugs had a lasting effect on her type 2 diabetes.

Cathy began by changing her eating habits: no snacking, no late-night eating, and only meals containing real whole foods. Within several weeks, her blood sugar levels came down and she was able to stop taking insulin. Several months later, she stopped taking metformin, and six months after she'd first started changing her diet, her insulin and fasting glucose were normal and she stopped the GLP-1. She'd reversed her type 2 diabetes.

More importantly, Cathy had developed new eating habits. Not only did she change what she ate but also when she ate it. The GLP-1 had helped her feel less hungry in the short term, but it didn't change her food habits or eating patterns. Learning about the hormonal response to food, fasting intermittently, and joining a community committed to long-term, sustainable weight loss did that. She's lost more than 100 pounds (45 kg), reduced her body and visceral fat, and has a new, healthy relationship with food.

HELEN

Helen was adopted at birth into a family of "naturally thin people" who could seemingly eat whatever they wanted. She, however, had always been heavier than average and felt a lot of guilt around eating. She'd come to believe that her excess weight and her chronic arthritis were her fault. At seventy-one, she'd had both shoulders replaced and was looking toward knee and hip replacements. She managed the pain with a steady diet of ibuprofen.

I immediately started Helen on a fasting protocol, to help lower her blood sugars and inflammation. Probably the most important lesson she learned was that weight gain isn't all about calories. To lose weight long term meant looking at the quality and quantity of food, the amount of daily exercise, and how to take care of herself emotionally and physically. She learned about her relationship with food and how her body works.

Helen has now reduced the amount of carbs she eats, uses a variety of fasting protocols, follows an eating and exercise schedule, and journals to keep track of and process her emotions around both of these issues. She's lost about 180 pounds (82 kg), walks 3.5 miles (5.6 km) every day, and plans to continue teaching for another ten years!

PART TWO

Hedonic Hunger

| 6 |

GETTING HOOKED ON
ULTRA-PROCESSED FOODS

N 2013, BRAZIL was facing a national crisis: obesity. Dr. Carlos Monteiro, an epidemiologist at the University of São Paulo, studying the data, noticed an odd paradox. People were buying less sugar, oil, and salt, but their weight was rising steadily. What else were they doing differently? They were swapping their traditional home-cooked foods for ready-to-eat foods like packaged cakes, cookies, breakfast cereals, crackers, potato chips, and sodas. As they did so, their weight went up. What did these foods have in common that was causing the rise in obesity?

In a word, ultra-processing. It wasn't the calories or the macronutrients (carbohydrates, proteins, fats) that defined these fattening foods. It was the ultra-processing. The packaged foods people were eating contained or were made using mostly highly processed ingredients, including artificial colors, flavors, and preservatives. An advisor to the World Health Organization, Dr. Monteiro worried that the different food groups of traditional dietary recommendations that focused on calories or macronutrient composition "muddle together fresh and minimally processed foods, processed ingredients, and ultra-processed products."

He concluded: "What should be said above all is that consumption—and production—of ultra-processed products needs to be minimized."[1] This conclusion was a revolutionary change.

In 2014, based on Dr. Monteiro's recommendation, the Brazilian government completely rewrote its dietary guidelines to concentrate on one action: getting its citizens to stop eating ultra-processed foods (UPFs). Dr. Monteiro and others believed this action was the single most important step for good health. This insight would ultimately transform the world of public health nutrition.

I had reached much the same conclusion in 2014 as I was writing *The Obesity Code*. In that book, I wrote: "Western diets are characterized by one defining feature—and it's not the amount of fat, salt, carbohydrate, or protein. It's the high amount of processing of foods." The problem is the processing. In the years since then, the scientific evidence has only grown stronger. Rather shockingly, UPFs have taken over 70 percent of the Standard American Diet and may be responsible for 21 percent of cases of obesity.[2] Over the past two decades alone, UPFs in the American diet have steadily grown across all ages, both sexes, and all demographic groups,[3] and the rest of the world is following close behind.

WHAT ARE ULTRA-PROCESSED FOODS?

IN EVERYDAY LANGUAGE, we talk about "junk food," "convenience food," and "fast food" to describe foods that are processed and packaged—and contribute to obesity. For foods that are in their original form, we say things like "natural foods," "raw foods," and "unprocessed foods." All those terms are imprecise from a scientific perspective. To better understand the differences between foods, Dr. Monteiro and his research group developed the NOVA food classification system. This system divides foods into four categories according to their level of processing (Figure 6.1[4]).[5]

Figure 6.1. The four groups of the NOVA food classification system, from unprocessed to ultra-processed foods

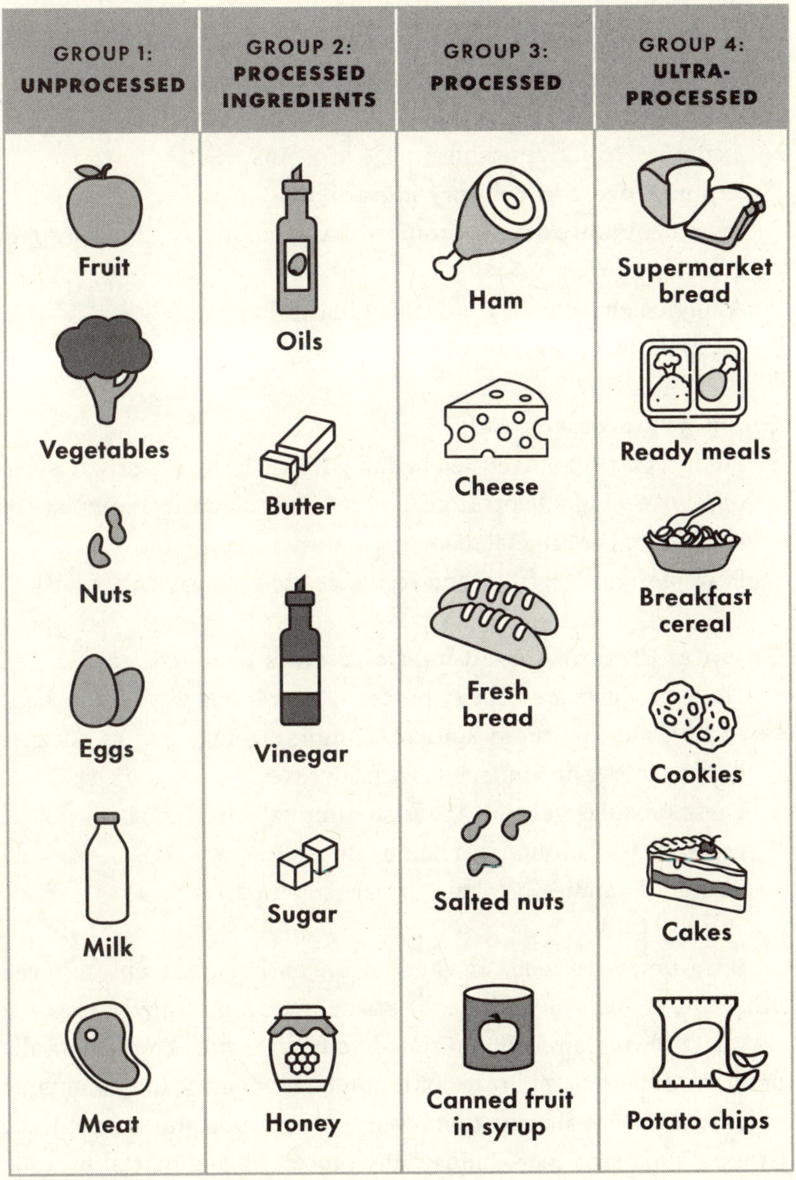

GROUP 1: UNPROCESSED	GROUP 2: PROCESSED INGREDIENTS	GROUP 3: PROCESSED	GROUP 4: ULTRA-PROCESSED
Fruit	Oils	Ham	Supermarket bread
Vegetables	Butter	Cheese	Ready meals
Nuts	Vinegar	Fresh bread	Breakfast cereal
Eggs	Sugar	Salted nuts	Cookies
Milk	Honey	Canned fruit in syrup	Cakes
Meat			Potato chips

101

Group 1: Unprocessed or minimally processed foods

- Plants or animals are obtained directly from nature and not altered following their removal from nature.
- Minimally processed foods are natural foods submitted only to cleaning, removing inedible parts, grinding, drying, fermenting, pasteurizing, cooling, or freezing.
  Examples: fruits, vegetables, meat, fish, nuts

Group 2: Processed culinary ingredients

- Ingredients are extracted from natural foods and used to season or cook foods.
- As ingredients, they are not usually eaten by themselves.
  Examples: salt, sugar, oils, honey, butter

Group 3: Processed foods

- Products are manufactured by industry with the use of salt, sugar, oil, or other ingredients from Group 2. They are easily recognized as versions of the original food.
  Examples: canned fruits and vegetables, tomato paste, beef jerky

Group 4: Ultra-processed food and drink products

- These products are usually processed in various ways from cheap, industrially produced sources, combining food basics such as dietary energy and nutrients with additives.
- These products generally contain minimal whole foods as well as ingredients not found in a home kitchen.
  Examples: candies, breakfast cereals, supermarket bread

Ultra-processed foods, in Group 4, are entirely different from the other three groups of foods because they are manufactured more than they are grown. Compare traditional homemade bread to industrially produced supermarket bread, for example. Homemade bread contains only flour, water, salt, sugar, and yeast, and is therefore classified as a Group 3 processed food. Industrially processed commercial bread is Group 4 since it also contains—from the ingredient list of a loaf of bread in my local store—calcium propionate, vegetable monoglycerides, sodium stearoyl-2-lactylate, sorbic acid, enzymes, and ascorbic acid, and may contain added wheat gluten, diacetyl tartaric acid esters of mono- and diglycerides, and L-cysteine hydrochloride.

Here is the ingredient list on another loaf of store-bought bread:

INGREDIENTS: enriched bleached flour (wheat flour, malted barley flour, niacin, reduced iron, thiamin mononitrate, riboflavin, folic acid), filtered water, durum wheat sourdough, contains 2% or less of: yeast, ascorbic acid, enzymes, sea salt, concentrated sponge extract wheat flour, cultured wheat flour.

What *is* this stuff? Concentrated sponge extract wheat flour? Cultured wheat flour? WTF? That's the point. If the food contains ingredients that you don't recognize, it's highly likely to be a UPF. Most store-bought bread, muffins, bagels, cakes, cookies, and biscuits fit squarely in the UPF category.

WHY ARE ULTRA-PROCESSED FOODS SO FATTENING?

UPFS CAN BE manipulated in almost infinite ways that natural or minimally processed foods cannot. Meat, for example, has only a certain range of proteins and fats. Milk is milk, no matter how much you want it to be different. Broccoli can be cooked in many ways but is still easily recognized as broccoli. UPFs, however, can be any percentage of fat or carbs or protein, taste like anything you want, and look like anything you want. You can make a UPF bigger or smaller. Heavier or lighter. Harder or softer. Savory or sweet. Think about a slice of commercial white bread or a cheese puff.

We know that controlling hunger is the key to weight loss. In 103 Chapter 5, we looked at the characteristics of satiating foods. Not accidentally, UPFs are created to be almost the exact opposite. Compare the differences (Table 6.1).

Table 6.1. The differences between satiating foods and ultra-processed foods

Characteristics of foods that create satiety, control hunger, and lead to weight loss	Characteristics of ultra-processed foods
Bulky—high volume and low energy density (full of fiber and water)	Small, with high energy density (reduces shipping costs)
Requires effort to chew and swallow	Very easy to chew and swallow (low bulk, protein, fiber, and water)
Natural, without additives	Many additives, to maximize eating pleasure (engineered to create maximum "bliss point")
High in protein	Low in protein
High in fiber	Very low in fiber
Low in sugar	High in sugar (cheap way to ramp up taste)
Low in processed fat	High in processed fats (natural fats are expensive; industrial seed oils are cheap)
Low Glycemic Index	High Glycemic Index (highly refined carbohydrates are cheap)
Heavy (create a feeling of weight in the stomach)	Very light (engineered for vanishing caloric density)
Naturally appealing	Artificially designed to be super-appealing (bright colors, fun shapes, heavily advertised)

We've already discussed some of these factors at length in previous chapters, so let's dive a little more into the other factors that make UPFs so dangerous.

UPFs are lower in protein

UPFs are often low in protein because it is more profitable for food manufacturers to replace protein with cheaper carbohydrates and add meat flavor and texture. Lower protein means less activation of satiety pathways like GLP-1 and peptide YY.

Even so-called high-protein UPFs start with cheap processed proteins like whey, which is a waste product of cheese-making, or soy or pea protein. Another example is creatine powder, which is touted for building muscle. Most people get creatine from eating seafood or red meat, but creatine powder is made by heating and pressurizing the chemicals sarcosine and cyanamide together to form creatine crystals that can be purified, dried, and milled. Not quite the high-quality beef steak most buyers of creatine powder have in mind.

Ultra-processed proteins may not have the same health effects as natural proteins like fish or eggs or meat. Think of the difference this way. Just because I'm a human doesn't mean I can play basketball like Michael Jordan, who is also a human.

UPFs are very low in fiber

UPFs are often created without fiber so they can be eaten quickly and easily. Commercial white bread, for example, often only has 1 to 2 grams of fiber per serving, whereas whole-grain bread might have five times that amount.

Removing fiber lowers bulk and weight from the final product. Low fiber means the stretch receptors in the stomach are not activated to signal satiety. Less fiber also means fewer short-chain fatty acids in the colon, which decreases satiety hormones such as GLP-1 and peptide YY.

UPFs have vanishing caloric density

Some UPFs barely need to be chewed; they seem to just melt in your mouth. Think about commercial white bread, cheese puffs, and potato chips. This phenomenon is called vanishing caloric density. Foods that are very light and easy to eat create almost no satiety, so it feels like you haven't eaten anything. Your body is tricked into believing that those calories have "vanished."

When natural foods are processed, their food matrix is disrupted. Grinding, cooking, steaming, emulsifying—all these processes break down the cell walls of plant and animal foods like a kind of "pre-digestion." Texturizers, common in making UPFs, are chemicals used to soften foods so they need less chewing. The point is to make it very easy to eat these foods and for the body to digest and absorb them quickly. As the rate of absorption increases, the feeling of fullness decreases. In other words, we eat more because we don't feel satiated. Even if we become satiated, we can easily eat UPFs well past this point because they are so "easy" to eat.

Very-easy-to-eat foods dodge our satiety mechanisms because our body needs time to register how full we are. Chewing and swallowing foods activates baroreceptors in our esophagus and stomach to let our brain know we are eating. When we are distracted, by watching TV or a movie, for example, or by looking at a computer screen or scrolling through social media, it is easy to mindlessly eat UPFs. We barely register that we are eating, and therefore we don't feel full. It's easy to devour a family-sized bag of potato chips or a box of cookies in front of the TV. You can put one UPF after another into your mouth and barely notice it. Try it with a bag of hard-to-chew carrot sticks. Not so easy.

Just look at your local grocery store. Entire aisles are filled with breakfast cereals, cookies, cakes, potato chips, corn chips, popcorn, pasta, prepared "side dishes," sodas, juices, and premade soups. Notice how all these foods follow the same playbook: low protein, low fiber, highly refined carbohydrates, with lots of added sugars and processed fats. This combination creates a low-bulk, light, easy-to-eat food that creates minimal satiety. It's a feature, not a design flaw. You eat more, so you buy more. *Cha-ching!*

The bottom line is that UPFs are artificially easy to eat and hyper-palatable, which means they are easy to

- eat and overeat,
- digest and absorb,
- wolf down,
- eat mindlessly, and
- become addicted to (more on this in Chapter 7).

Do UPFs make you fat? Hell yes.

On a nutrition label, a sugary cereal can look the same as a bean salad. Yet these two foods are very different in their hormonal response and their health effects. An influential 2019 study emphasized the out-sized role of UPFs in obesity.[6] Twenty participants ate either minimally processed foods or UPFs. Both diets contained the same nutrients (sugar, fat, protein, sodium, carbohydrates, and fiber), and participants were allowed to eat as much or as little as they liked for the fourteen days of each diet. What happened?

The people eating the UPF diet

- ate about 500 calories more per day;
- ate about 40 percent faster;
- ate more carbs and fats, and about the same levels of protein;
- gained 3 pounds (1.4 kg) more weight;
- showed increased insulin effect, as measured by C-peptide;
- showed increased respiratory quotient (indicating the body is mostly burning carbs); and
- burned about 171 extra calories per day.

The UPF diet maximized hunger, minimized satiety, and increased the insulin effect. No wonder people gained weight! The body sensed this increase in food and tried to burn off more sugar (carbs) and calories, but this homeostatic mechanism was not enough to reverse the weight gain. The UPFs simply overwhelmed the body fat thermostat (Figure 6.2).

Figure 6.2. Ultra-processed food decreases satiety but increases hunger and insulin, which makes us gain weight

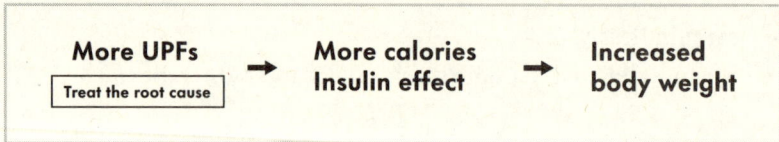

More UPFs Treat the root cause	→	More calories Insulin effect	→	Increased body weight

Here's the important thing. The biggest problem is not the calories or fat or protein or carbs. It is the **level of processing**. The increase in calories and carbohydrates and body weight are symptoms. The root cause of weight gain is that ultra-processing causes people to eat more calories, more carbs, and more fat.

For lasting success, you need to treat the root cause (the ultra-processed foods), not the proximate cause or symptom (the increase in calories, carbs, insulin, and body weight). If you have depression that causes alcoholism, then you must treat the depression. You don't need to be told to "Drink less alcohol" because it's an "alcohol balance problem."

But this exact same logic is always given for weight loss. Eat fewer calories. But if the UPFs caused people to eat more calories in the first place, then the best advice is to "Eat fewer UPFs" rather than "Eat fewer calories."

What is the point of bioengineering UPFs to be super-low-satiety foods? Money, money, money. Food companies make more money when they sell more food. If the food they sell doesn't make you full, you'll eat more. Then you'll buy more and they'll make more money. The unfortunate (for you) side effect is that you'll get fat. The food company doesn't care. They can always blame you for low willpower. They can always fall back on the Calories In, Calories Out argument. They can always tell you to exercise more. No wonder weight loss can be such an uphill battle.

HOW DID ULTRA-PROCESSED FOODS TAKE OVER THE WORLD?

TODAY, THE ULTRA-FATTENING UPFs have almost completely displaced minimally processed foods to dominate America's diet. From 1800 to 2019, UPFs grew from less than 5 percent of the calories Americans eat to over 60 percent.[7] While the United States has the largest proportion of its diet provided by UPFs, many other nations in the world are catching up quickly. For generations, the foods people ate would have been mostly natural ones, knowledge of them handed down from generation to generation, cooked in the traditional methods of culture and place. Food traditions do change over time, but, at least until 1977, they did so relatively slowly.

The U.S. government's *Dietary Goals for the United States* of 1977 set the direction for what Americans would eat for decades to come. The guidelines focused on nutrients (calories, carbs, fats, and proteins) rather than foods (broccoli, fish, eggs), yet a nutrient only describes a single factor in the food. The government zeroed in on dietary fat, but dozens of other characteristics (weight, texture, volume, added chemical flavorings, emulsifiers, softness, food matrix, fiber, acidity, ease of digestion, bitterness, sweetness, Glycemic Index, to name but a few) influence the body's hormonal and satiety responses.

In one fell swoop, all these other factors were unconsciously declared to be largely irrelevant. A healthy diet, they counseled, was all about calories. Americans were eating too many calories, and fat was the culprit. Overnight, we went from eating natural foods containing fat, such as beef, avocados, dairy, and fish, to being told we should eat low-fat everything. You've heard it a million times: "a calorie is a calorie." This model is simple, easy to understand, **and completely wrong**. How natural a food was, how much processing a food underwent, how a food was prepared, all became irrelevant in the obsessive focus on calories and macronutrients (fat, carbohydrates, and proteins). The consequences were disastrous.

The new dietary guidelines changed the way most of us eat, allowing ultra-processed foods, like a Trojan horse, to sneak into and overwhelm the American diet. Converting natural foods into low-fat foods required ultra-processing in a factory. When you take fat out of food, the flavor of those foods suffers. So food companies began to replace the fat with a lot of sugar, but also emulsifiers, texturizers, artificial flavors, and artificial colors to maintain taste and mouthfeel. In essence, the government declared (without any scientific evidence, it turns out), that it is better to eat low-fat fake foods compared to higher-fat natural foods. For generations, dieticians and doctors parroted this party line. Low fat? Mission accomplished. Healthy? Not even a little.

The hidden mega-profit opportunity soon revealed itself. Ultra-processed low-fat foods could claim the halo of health benefits, but more importantly, they could be trademarked as branded products that other companies couldn't reproduce. Unlike natural foods, UPFs are made exclusively by for-profit companies and can be trademarked and "owned." Nobody could trademark broccoli or cheddar cheese, but Cheetos? Absolutely. Homemade bread was out. Packaged, sliced Wonder Bread was in.

Governments and scientists loved it. Low-fat, low-calorie foods were defined as healthy, so who cared if those foods were completely artificial and ultra-processed? The American Heart Association sold their Heart-Check mark, endorsing many, many ultra-processed foods like sugary cereals as "heart healthy." UPFs flooded into the supermarkets disguised as "health foods" because foods were considered equal if the calories and macronutrients (carbs, proteins, and fats) were equivalent. Cookies were the same as quinoa. Hot dogs were the same as salmon. Sugary cereals were the same as apples. This belief was a godsend to the processed-food industry.

110

If you lived through the 1980s, you'll remember the low-fat UPF mania, along with skinny ties, big hair, and the (shudder) power ballad.

Baked potato chips. Diet sodas. Low-fat yogurts. Low-fat processed meats. Turkey… everything. Carb loading. Low-fat candies. Pretzels were in. Beef jerky was out. Lean Cuisine. Crystal Light. Healthy Choice. Fat-free frozen yogurt. Fat-free baked goods. Fat-free salad dressings. Sports drinks. I Can't Believe It's Not Butter!

I Can't Believe We Ate That Crap.

In 1989, 626 new reduced-fat foods were introduced to market, up an eye-popping 127 percent from the year prior.[8] In 1994, SnackWell's, a brand of no-fat cookies which tasted only a tiny bit better than cardboard, topped the cookie charts after a mere two years on the market, displacing decades of dominance by the humbled Oreo. Low-fat diet foods were a juggernaut rampaging through the 1980s and 1990s.

Did anybody lose weight? Hell no. Americans gained weight faster than any other time in U.S. history. But the profits in manufactured foods sure went up. The value of companies that manufacture UPFs grew exponentially during the 1980s and has never looked back (Figure 6.3[9]).[10]

Figure 6.3. The value of companies manufacturing UPFs climbed significantly after 1977

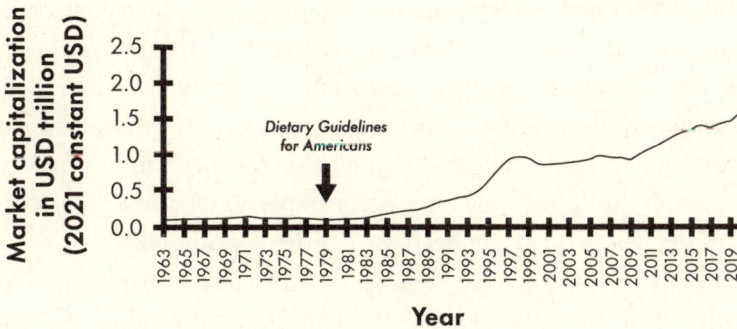

Ultra-processed foods aren't just popular with the brand manufacturers. Consumers love them. In our busy modern world, it's hard to overlook the fact that ultra-processed foods are cheaper and more convenient than natural foods. They have a long shelf life. They are engineered to be flavorful in ways that natural foods are not. UPFs are designed to appeal to us on every level. Too bad about that whole "gaining weight" thing.

THE ADVANTAGES OF ULTRA-PROCESSING

ULTRA-PROCESSED FOODS, like the iconic sliced white bread, have many advantages over natural, unprocessed foods. Not only are they super easy to eat, and eat quickly, but they are

- cheap,
- tasty and good-looking,
- convenient and shelf-stable,
- endlessly variable,
- easy to market/advertise, and
- super-profitable due to industrial processing and scale.

With all these advantages over real foods, who can resist?

UPFs are cheap

In the 1950s, households spent about 32 percent of their household budget on food.[11] Today, that's down to about 13 percent.[12] Why? UPFs, baby. They are much, much cheaper than minimally processed foods. The price per calorie drops 8.7 percent for every 10 percent increase in processing.[13] For some categories of food, that number is more dramatic. For example, for soups and stews, every 10 percent increase in processing results in a 24.3 percent decrease in price per calorie.

UPFs are cheap because they start with cheap ingredients like heavily subsidized crops of corn, wheat, and soy. Ultra-processing and chemical additives do the rest of the work. Artificial flavors can make them taste however manufacturers want. Texturizers, emulsifiers, and modified starches can give UPFs any type of mouthfeel. Artificial colors can make UPFs look like anything. A UPF might be cheap, but it looks and tastes expensive.

The wide availability of cheap UPFs explains why poverty and obesity are so closely intertwined. If you don't have much money to spend on food, you can stretch your budget by eating UPFs that taste very close to the original foods. Instead of eating whole ingredients and whole foods, you get cheap industrial ingredients with chemicals to add taste, texture, and flavor that make you fat. But hey, the price is right.

UPFs are tasty and look good

UPFs look like real foods. Consider sour cream and its UPF doppelgänger. Natural sour cream has only one ingredient: cultured cream. Near my house, only one of five grocery stores sells this natural product. The rest sell a UPF sour cream that contains whey, modified corn starch, gelatin, sodium phosphate, guar gum, carrageenan, sodium citrate, calcium sulfate, and locust bean gum. Seriously. What the hell? The point is that cream is expensive, so it's much, much cheaper to use whey, gelatin, modified starches, and other chemicals (carrageenan and so on) to make this product taste almost exactly like sour cream.

Or consider McDonald's french fries. Once upon a time, they consisted of potatoes deep-fried in a natural fat—beef tallow—and salt. On its website in 2024, McDonald's listed the following ingredients for its fries:

> Potatoes, Vegetable Oil (Canola Oil, Corn Oil, Soybean Oil, Hydrogenated Soybean Oil, Natural Beef Flavor [Wheat and Milk Derivatives]*), Dextrose, Sodium Acid Pyrophosphate (maintain Color), Salt.
> *Natural Beef Flavor Contains Hydrolyzed Wheat and Hydrolyzed Milk as Starting Ingredients.
> Contains: Wheat, Milk.

113

Seriously. McDonald's french fries contained wheat and milk. The potatoes, colored with sodium acid pyrophosphate to look like french fries, are really only there to hold the "beef flavor." And why would "natural" beef flavor start with hydrolyzed wheat and milk?

The answer is money, money, money. Why use expensive real ingredients when you can use cheap, industrial chemicals? The UPF will still taste pretty much the same as the natural food. Why use real vanilla for several hundred dollars per pound when you can use vanillin, a synthetic chemical that tastes like vanilla for about ten dollars per pound? Vanillin is one of the most common chemical additives in UPFs. Why use real strawberry when you can use ethyl methylphenylglycidate with some modified starches and other chemicals to mimic the texture, flavor, and aroma of strawberry?

UPFs are convenient and shelf-stable

UPFs maximize convenience. They come in a package—like a box, a bag, or a microwaveable tray that you can throw in the cupboard or the freezer until you need it. Sometimes, you can even use the packaging to cook the foods. UPFs have a long shelf life and some seem to never spoil. They are consistent. Every product is exactly the same, so no risk of sour grapes or rotten apples. Every Twinkie is identical. If they're not ready to eat, UPFs can be made quickly and with a minimum of effort—sometimes just adding water. And they are easily available, not only at the supermarket, but also in convenience stores and vending machines.

UPFs are endlessly variable

Variety is the spice of life. Unfortunately, this fact also makes you overeat. Monotonous diets are great for weight loss because when we eat the same thing all the time, we get tired of it. This phenomenon is called sensory-specific satiety. Once your homeostatic hunger is sated, you'll stop eating because eating is not particularly pleasurable. If you ate white rice and boiled vegetables for every meal for several decades, then the next meal of rice and vegetables wouldn't excite you much.

Broccoli is broccoli. Beef is beef. Yes, you can cook them in different ways, but that hardly compares to the virtually infinite number of ways to prepare UPFs. Consider potato chips. Yes, there is regular flavor, but there is also sour cream and onion, bacon, ketchup, dill pickle—even fancy flavors like truffle, kimchi, and curry. There's thick cut and thin cut. There's waffle cut. Or consider donuts. Yes, there are plain donuts, but there are dozens of frosting flavors available. There are thousands of chemical flavoring agents, coloring agents, emulsifying agents, and so on. If you can imagine the flavor, someone can create it. The variations are unlimited.

When even a mild variation is available, we get hungry again. Our brains are wired to respond to both new experiences and complex flavors, likely to encourage us to eat a wide variety of foods so that we get all the various nutrients we need. If we eat broccoli all the time, we don't want more. In contrast, UPFs can present us with unlimited variety, causing unlimited hunger.

UPFs are easy to market and advertise

You don't see many ads for broccoli. Or salmon. There are thousands of farmers growing broccoli and thousands of people who fish, but they don't advertise because nobody "owns" the name. They don't employ large marketing departments with advertising budgets and summer interns. UPFs are owned and trademarked and manufactured by companies, not grown or harvested. The brand, whether Oreos or Cheetos or Froot Loops, and its owner benefit directly from advertising and are therefore heavily marketed. In weekly supermarket ads, UPFs constitute almost half of the products advertised.[14]

UPFs are packaged with vivid, enticing logos in bright colors and with carefully crafted messages like "8 essential vitamins and minerals." They are advertised on TV with catchy jingles. Companies pay to get prime shelf space for these products in the supermarket. And these same companies spend a lot of their advertising budget targeting children with movie placements and cartoon character endorsements. By contrast, broccoli always looks like broccoli. Meat like meat. Fish like fish. Real food just can't compete with the ubiquitous UPF advertising.

UPFs are super-profitable

UPFs are manufactured cheaply with economies of scale, branded, and then mass marketed. This industrialization and commercialization maximizes profits. The UPF ingredients can be carefully adjusted to find the ultimate "bliss point" to maximize sales. Finding that point means making sure you eat more, you eat quickly, and you eat the product again and again. The downside is that UPFs make you fat and unhealthy. But, hey! That's not the food company's problem. That's *your* problem.

Despite our best efforts to protect them from manipulative advertising practices, children are heavily affected by the messaging. The average Canadian three-year-old child gets a stunning 45 percent of their calories from ultra-processed foods. Every 10 percent increase in UPF consumption is associated with a 17 percent increase in the risk of being overweight or obese at age five.[15]

THE FIRST GOLDEN RULE:
AVOID ULTRA-PROCESSED FOODS

The Golden Rule of the Brazilian dietary guideline is: "Always prefer natural or minimally processed foods and freshly made dishes and meals to ultra-processed foods."[16] Part of the genius of this guiding principle is that it provides clear, unambiguous advice and avoids complicated food rules. And because UPFs affect obesity on so many different levels, this rule to avoid UPFs to the maximum extent possible is perhaps the most important food rule of all. Food writer Michael Pollan captured its essence in his book *Food Rules* by urging us to "Eat food" rather than "edible food-like substances."[17]

Real food is unprocessed. Real food has a simple ingredient list. Real food isn't advertised on TV. Real food would be recognizable to your great-grandmother. Real food is cooked by real humans.

But there is hope yet, as UPFs have not completely taken over the world. The Italian diet, for example, consists of less than 10 percent UPFs.[18] Perhaps not coincidentally, the rate of obesity in Italy is about 12 percent (compared to almost 42 percent in the U.S.),[19,20] despite their famous love of food and pasta.

The best way to not eat UPFs is to become aware of them so you don't bring them into your home where you will be tempted to eat them. At the grocery store, shop the perimeter where you generally find the fruits, vegetables, eggs, dairy, meat, and fish. That's not a fool-proof method for avoiding UPFs, however. Here are two tips:

1. get to know the most common UPFs and
2. avoid food with labels.

Take this list of common UPFs with you the next time you go to the grocery store or order food online.

Get to know the most common UPFs

These most common UPFs eaten in the Western diet[21] will come as no surprise, but minimizing the foods on this list is a great place to start.[22]

- Factory-made white bread (11% of calories in typical diet)
  - Wonder Bread, sandwich slices, buns, toast, cornbread, croissants, bagels, wraps, crumpets, banana bread, baguettes, rolls, pita, tortilla, bread sticks
- Pre-packaged meals (8%)
  - Boxed macaroni and cheese, instant noodles, frozen pizza and other frozen meals, fish sticks, chicken nuggets
- Breakfast cereals (4%)
- Sausages and other reconstituted meat products (4%)
- Candies, chocolates, and snacks (4%)
  - Energy bars, granola bars, sweetened or colored fruit leather
- Biscuits (4%)
  - Cookies, crackers, wafers
- Store-bought bakery products (3%)
- cakes, rolls, buns, wraps, muffins, mixes, waffles, pancakes, cones, cupcakes, donuts, pie, pastries, stuffing
- Factory-made chips and fries (3%)
- Soft drinks, fruit drinks, and fruit juices (3%)
- Salty snacks (2%)
  - potato chips, corn chips, cheese puffs
- Sauces, dressings, and gravy (2%)
  - Commercial salad dressings, ketchup, instant sauces
- Instant soups, powdered soups
- Margarine, most spreads
- Processed cheese (just yuck)
  - Includes products made with "milk protein concentrate," which include artificial colors and flavors that mimic the look and taste of cheese

Certain chemicals and ingredients are used exclusively in UPFs. These dodgy ingredients are reliable markers for UPFs.

- Anti-caking agents
- Anti-foaming agents
- Artificial colors
- Artificial flavors or "flavor enhancers"—for example, monosodium glutamate

- Emulsifiers, emulsifying agents, emulsifying salts
- Gelling and glazing agents, such as guar gum, xanthan gum, tapioca starch, agar
- Hydrogenated or inter-esterified oil
- Hydrolyzed proteins, soya protein isolates, casein, whey protein, mechanically separated meat
- Modified starches—mostly cheap filler to add bulk to foods. Modified starches can thicken, change mouthfeel, hold on to batter easier, resist freezer burn, and so on. An average consumer eats about 30 pounds (13.6 kg) of modified starches every year without ever knowing it.
- Silicon dioxide, calcium silicate, magnesium stearate
- Seed oils. Natural fats are expensive and industrial seed oils are cheap. A food that contains palm, corn, soybean, vegetable, canola, safflower, or sunflower oil has a greater than 80 percent chance of being a UPF.[23]
- Sugars/sweeteners by other names—invert sugar, malto-dextrin, dextrose, lactose, high-fructose corn syrup, fruit juice concentrate
- Thickeners, bulking agents
- Unrecognizable ingredients—for example, calcium propionate

Take extra care with the following dodgy ingredients, which are available in the U.S. but limited or banned in most of Canada, Europe, the U.K., Australia, and New Zealand.

- Artificial food dyes
- Astaxanthin—found in farm-raised salmon to make flesh pink
- Brominated vegetable oil—found in many citrus-flavored sodas
- Butylated hydroxyanisole (BHA)—preservative found in cereals, baked goods, and snacks
- Butylated hydroxytoluene (BHT)—preservative found in many breakfast cereals, frozen foods, prepared snacks, dried and processed meats
- Genetically modified foods
- High-fructose corn syrup
- Potassium bromate—found in commercial factory-made bread
- Recombinant bovine growth hormone (rBGH)—used in U.S. dairy to increase milk production
- Trans fats

THE TRULY SAD PART is that compiling this list of dubious ingredients only took a quick trip to my local grocery store. These UPFs have infiltrated our lives so completely that we don't even notice them anymore.

Avoid foods with labels

The well-meaning advice to read food labels is probably good advice, but not in the way that most people think. If the food you're buying has a food label, then you probably shouldn't be eating that food. What is on the label hardly matters; it likely won't be good. Natural foods— meat, fish, eggs, vegetables, fruits, and so on—usually don't have food labels. If they do, the label should list three or fewer ingredients on it, and your grandmother should be able to recognize all of them. The rest of the information on the food label—calories, carbohydrates, proteins, and so on—has limited value for weight loss.

Remember that foods contain both energy (calories) and information (instructions for hormonal response). UPFs are incredibly effective at making people gain weight because they affect *both* how many calories we eat and how the hormones (insulin, GLP-1, stomach baroreceptors, among others) of our homeostatic hunger system respond. When we eat natural, unprocessed foods, our hunger is limited by satiety. UPFs circumvent this homeostatic hunger.

But the news gets worse. In addition to the physiological responses we've discussed, UPFs stimulate the brain reward centers. And just as UPFs cause our physical body to want more, they also cause our brain to desire more. That combination opens the door to a proven method of supercharging profitability. Nothing feeds profits like selling addiction.

| 7 |

UNDERSTANDING
FOOD ADDICTION

I N THE 1800S, the British East India Company smuggled narcotics from India into China to turn citizens into addicts, eventually leading to the Opium Wars. That's the kind of ruthlessness that wins you a global empire. Today, drug lords in many parts of the world profit heavily by selling illicit, addictive drugs like cocaine and heroin.

That strategy is even more profitable when the addictive product is legal. Alcohol companies generate enormous profits while alcoholism generates enormous social harms. The tobacco industry reaps billions while the average smoker incurs US$86,001 to $194,899 over their lifetime in out-of-pocket costs.[1] Drinking and smoking might seem cool, but it's actually the addictive nature of alcohol and nicotine that keeps users coming back.

Addiction is also the key to big profits in technology. A shocking 43 percent of Americans consider themselves addicted to their cell phone, checking it an average of 205 times per day.[2] But another addictive product may rule them all: ultra-processed foods.

CAN FOODS REALLY BE ADDICTIVE?

ADDICTION CAN BE defined as a repetitive behavior that some people find difficult to quit. Not everyone must develop a problem for a substance to be addictive. Alcohol and tobacco are addictive, yet many people drink or smoke occasionally without becoming addicted. The same is true with food.

Certain areas in our brain (reward centers) create pleasurable feelings to reward good behaviors. When we enjoy activities—meeting friends, playing games or sports, eating foods we like, for example—feel-good chemicals in the brain, called neurotransmitters, are released. These neurotransmitters include dopamine, serotonin, and endorphins. Because we feel good, we do these activities again and again.

Drugs with addictive potential, such as cocaine and alcohol, also target these neurotransmitter reward centers. In fact, many substances and many activities can be addictive. The difference between normal pleasurable behaviors and addictive ones depends primarily on three factors:

1. Supernormal stimulation
2. Neurotransmitter spike
3. Availability (cost/accessibility/marketing)

Supernormal stimulation

Supernormal stimuli are exaggerated versions of normal stimuli that elicit a stronger reaction than the original. For example, in one experiment, birds given a larger, brighter fake egg to guard preferred it to their own natural pale eggs. Sometimes these fake eggs were so monstrously large that the birds slid off them, yet the birds persisted in guarding the eggs. In other experiments, colorful dummy butterflies have been found to attract more male attention than natural female butterflies. These stimuli are specifically designed to catch our attention.

Addictive drugs can deliver a supernormal stimulus that naturally pleasurable experiences cannot. The body produces natural endorphins, but that feel-good dose of endorphins is tiny compared to the "high" produced by cocaine or other illicit drugs. Alcohol is present naturally in small amounts in some fermented fruits, but it is hardly enough to create a buzz like the more concentrated quantities in a bottle of whiskey.

The same holds true for foods. Eating sweet foods stimulates dopamine release. Natural foods have a limit on their sweetness and how much dopamine is released. UPFs do not. For example, the natural sweetness of a strawberry is pleasant but limited: a one-cup bowl of strawberries contains around 7 grams of sugar. You can't increase the natural sweetness of the strawberry. In contrast, a one-cup bowl of sugary cereal can contain over 50 percent sugar, or 17 grams. This sugary cereal produces a supersized dopamine spike that natural foods cannot compete with. Like illicit drugs, processing is the key to concentrating the addictive substance.

Sugar isn't the only food additive that can boost a normal pleasurable experience to an addictive one. Other additives can stimulate a supersized dopamine spike too:

- Artificial sweeteners—sugar replacements that may confuse the brain's reward system
- Emulsifiers (soy lecithin, mono- and diglycerides)—substances that enhance mouthfeel
- High-fructose corn syrup (HFCS)—a sugar that enhances sweetness and may disrupt hormones like ghrelin, leading to increased food cravings
- Maltodextrin and other sugar derivatives—sugars that add unlimited sweetness
- Monosodium glutamate (MSG)—a flavor enhancer to boost umami
- Natural and artificial flavors—flavor enhancers
- Salt—a flavor enhancer to boost the intensity of flavors in food

The exact combination of these additives and how much of each to add to a product is typically optimized with focus groups. How much salt can you add before it starts to detract from the palatability? How much sugar? How much fat? Nothing is left to chance.

Natural foods cannot deliver a supernormal stimulus, and therefore their addictive potential is low. On the other hand, UPFs are designed to maximize the pleasurable experience, which may cross the line into addiction.

Neurotransmitter spike

Dopamine normally rises and falls in a controlled manner. We may go to a party and remember it fondly afterward. We might go for a run and feel good for a few hours after. We might listen to music we like and feel uplifted. In all of these cases, dopamine gradually rises and then fades. This effect is normal and we do not become addicted. When dopamine suddenly spikes very high and very quickly, it creates an unnaturally intense pleasure and the addictive potential surges.

To spike dopamine, a drug must be ingested and absorbed very, very quickly. Highly addictive drugs such as heroin or cocaine are usually injected intravenously, inhaled, or smoked so that a very high dose is delivered directly into the bloodstream. The ensuing "high" is intense enough to cause cravings and addiction. Smoking tobacco quickly spikes nicotine levels because of the high dose delivered to the bloodstream, whereas nicotine gum or patches release nicotine much more slowly and are far less addictive. This slow release helps people wean off smoking.

Foods that are ingested and absorbed quickly spike dopamine in the same way. Natural foods are embedded within a food matrix whose physical structure slows down the absorption of glucose and other nutrients. But UPFs disrupt this food matrix to accelerate the rate at which glucose is ingested, digested, and absorbed. UPFs are very soft and very easy to eat, sometimes dissolving on contact. A puffed cereal or snack, for example, has had its fiber and protein removed, and the resulting carbohydrate ground into a fine dust. By delivering glucose into the blood super-quickly, the UPF creates a massive spike in glucose, insulin, and dopamine. The power, potency, and speed of the

124

food-reward "high" delivered to our brain is completely unnatural. Yet the "hyper-palatable" combination of fat, sugar, salt, and/or carbs is particularly appealing to the brain's reward system, which makes such foods hard to resist.

Availability

Addictive substances become more harmful if they are cheap, easily accessible, heavily marketed, and socially acceptable. Alcohol, for example, is estimated to be three times more harmful to society than cocaine[3] due to its easy availability. Tobacco has become more expensive (due to taxes), less accessible, less marketed, and less socially acceptable, so its overall health risk has diminished. (But recently we've seen an increase in the number of people vaping nicotine because it is cheap, easily accessible in a wide variety of flavors, heavily marketed toward young adults, and more socially acceptable than smoking.) Cocaine is expensive, hard to access, not marketed, and not socially acceptable. This fact decreases its addictive potential over the general population.

UPFs have the highest potential for harm given their ubiquity in the modern diet. UPFs are cheaper, more easily accessible, more heavily marketed, and more socially acceptable than any other addictive substance by a wide, wide margin. This is a problem.

At first glance, the idea of foods being addictive seems like a stretch. Foods are all natural! However, upon reflection, this logic does not hold. Almost all addictive substances are derived from natural ingredients. Alcohol is fermented from barley, grains, potatoes, and so on. Nicotine is derived from tobacco plants. Marijuana is derived from the cannabis plant. Opium and its narcotic derivatives morphine and heroin are derived from poppies. It is the *processing* that transforms natural substances into addictive ones.

The addicting substance (alcohol, nicotine, cannabis) is concentrated and enhanced with other chemicals (sugar with alcohol or menthol with nicotine). The same holds true for foods. A natural food such as corn is not particularly addictive. Through ultra-processing,

125

the starch is purified, concentrated, ground up for quick absorption, mixed with flavorful additives to enhance the rewarding experience, and, voilà!, you have a highly addictive cheese puff. The very quick dopamine "hit" is potentially addictive.

Creating addictive UPFs is quite straightforward. Supersize the dose of sugar and refined carbohydrates (supernormal stimulation). Speed up absorption by removing protein, fiber, bulk, and weight (neurotransmitter spike). Add other flavors (salt, fats, artificial flavors) to increase the appeal. Make the product convenient, cheap, accessible—and advertise the hell out of it, especially to children (availability). Buy some biased research or make some dubious health claims for good measure. Who better to take advantage of that opportunity than Big Tobacco?

HOW BIG TOBACCO COMPANIES
HELPED MAKE UPFS ADDICTIVE

AFTER THE U.S. Surgeon General first warned about the dangers of smoking in 1964, public perception of tobacco slowly but inexorably changed. First came the bans on smoking in public places. Then came the warning labels on cigarette packages and restrictions on tobacco advertising. Smoking went from "cool" to "disgusting and filthy," even among the cool kids. The links to cancer, heart disease, and stroke were too strong to ignore. Whereas half of Canadians smoked in the 1960s, that number fell to less than a third by the 1990s.[4] The easy money in tobacco was over.

Big Tobacco companies had begun to look for other ways to leverage their prowess with manipulating flavors, marketing products, lobbying politicians, and influencing scientists. The natural successor was ultra-processed foods. In 1985, R.J. Reynolds Tobacco Company bought food giant Nabisco. The same year, tobacco giant Philip Morris (now Altria) bought processed food giant General Foods and then added Kraft in 1988. It was time to dust off the Big Tobacco "How to Sell an Addiction" playbook.

Step 1: Market to kids

Big Tobacco understood the power of advertising to children, the most susceptible segment of our population. Joe Camel, a cartoon mascot for Camel cigarettes, was an advertising legend, making cigarettes fun and appealing to children and high school students. Researchers found, for example, that in the three years after the cartoon character was introduced, "Camel's share of the illegal children's cigarette market segment increased from 0.5% to 32.8%,"[5] worth a cool US$476 million per year. An incredible 91.3 percent of six-year-old children in 1991 recognized Joe Camel and the Camel brand of cigarettes.[6]

After Big Tobacco acquired food brands, that marketing expertise was applied to UPFs like sugary breakfast cereals. Soon cereal boxes abounded with lovable cartoon characters—from mascots like the colorful Toucan Sam to Tony the Tiger to today's characters from cartoon movie tie-ins (*Cars, Shrek, Toy Story,* and so on). Children's TV channels are overrun with ads for UPFs. In the United States, almost $14 billion is spent per year on food advertising, and about 80 percent of that total promotes fast food, sugary drinks, unhealthy snacks, and candy.[7]

Advertising to children carries several important benefits, even when those products (tobacco) are specifically banned for minors. First, children form lifelong positive associations with the product and brand and become lifelong customers. Second, children are particularly susceptible to suggestion as they are still forming their personalities and preferences. Third, children's attitudes may rub off on older siblings and parents.

Step 2: Capture science and scientists

The next step to creating a national addiction is to bias research findings and influence doctors and other scientists. This scientific capture occurs when powerful actors—often corporations—influence or control scientific research to support their profits or market position. The tactics are varied, but the results are the same: generating "science" that favors whatever the brand is selling.

To legitimize smoking in the 1980s, Philip Morris implemented its secret Whitecoat Project whose goal was to "generate a body of scientific and technical knowledge" to "restore social acceptability of smoking."[8] Essentially, they paid doctors to publish ghostwritten studies to make it look like smoking and secondhand smoke were harmless. This deception would be uncovered during litigation involving tobacco firms, but not before its lessons were applied to UPFs.

Almost everybody agrees that we should eat less sugar. So it appears bizarre that some doctors promote sugar like it's a health food. It's less bizarre once you realize that their endorsement of sugar was bought and paid for, and that this arrangement has been going on for decades. In the 1960s, the Sugar Association, the trade association for the sugar industry in the U.S., paid Harvard researchers to disparage the link between sugar and heart disease in favor of cholesterol and fat in the prestigious *New England Journal of Medicine*.[9] Independently funded studies invariably find that sugar-sweetened beverages are linked to obesity, but 95.2 percent of studies funded by the Sugar Association have found no association.[10] The "scientific" results are based almost entirely on who pays the researchers. University of Toronto researchers received hundreds of thousands of dollars from industry groups, as reported in 2015.[11]

Similarly, in 2015, the University of Colorado School of Medicine was forced to return $1 million to the Coca-Cola Company earmarked to establish the Global Energy Balance Network (GEBN). The network blamed a lack of exercise—rather than sugary drinks and junk food—for America's burgeoning obesity problem.[12] Dr. Marion Nestle, a professor of nutrition and public health advocate, called the GEBN a "front group." This GEBN money was no one-off payment. Coke was forced to admit that it had given over $120 million between 2010 and 2015 to various academic institutions.

Big Tobacco companies have made UPFs widely available and marketed them heavily. They have targeted their advertising to children, knowing that parents want to make their kids happy, and they have promoted the health benefits of their products, knowing that most of us want to do things that help rather than harm our bodies. The result is that UPFs are embedded everywhere: in our school cafeterias, community center vending machines, and grocery stores. By 2016, UPFs provided about 60 percent of the diet, and almost 90 percent of the added sugars in a typical American diet. UPFs contain almost ten times more added sugars (21.1% of calories) compared to merely processed foods (2.4% of calories).[13]

Is food addiction a real problem? As real as a getting punched in the face. In 2015, almost 92 percent of people indicated some element of food addiction.[14] More recently, the Yale Food Addiction Scale (YFAS) has rigorously defined the syndrome of food addiction, and an estimated 14 percent of adults and 12 percent of children experience food addiction, a rate of addiction similar to alcohol (14%) and tobacco (18%). The numbers are sobering.[15] However, the recognition of this syndrome lags far behind, although scientific research has exploded since 2010 as evidenced by the exponential rise in recent publications (Figure 7.1[16]).[17]

Figure 7.1. The number of publications citing food addiction has grown exponentially since 2010

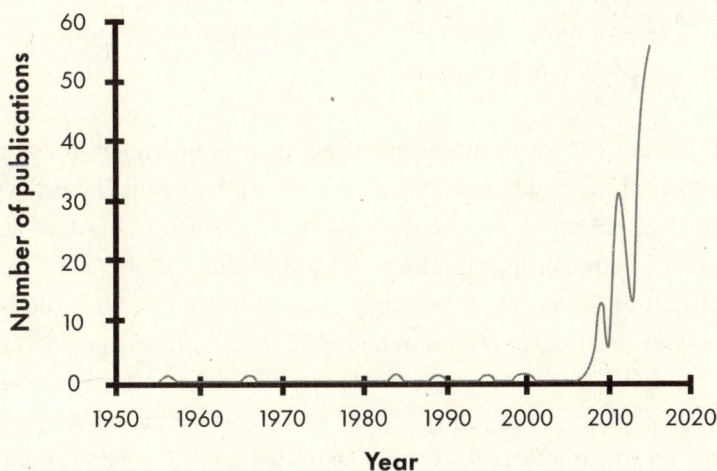

For people with excess weight, food addiction is even more common. It is estimated to affect 18 to 25 percent of people whose body mass index falls into the overweight or obese category compared to only 11.1 percent in people of normal weight.[18] Other highly affected groups include people with binge eating (57.6%),[19] those considering bariatric surgery (32%), and people with type 2 diabetes (30%).[20]

As you might expect, people with food addiction have more trouble losing weight.[21] They showed higher activation of the reward pathways on functional magnetic resonance imaging (fMRI). Importantly, the patterns of activation in response to food in "food addicts" is not fundamentally different than with other drugs of abuse.[22]

WHICH FOODS ARE ADDICTIVE?

THE EARLIEST SCIENTIFIC descriptions of food addiction appeared in 1956, identifying foods that "as a result of processing, come to have a materially changed rate of absorption."[23] Highly addictive foods share some common traits:

1. They are ultra-processed.
2. They have a high glycemic load or Glycemic Index.
3. They combine refined carbohydrates + fats.
4. They contain other flavors.

Glycemic load and Index are direct measurements of how quickly foods are absorbed. Therefore, foods with low Glycemic Index have low addictive potential. For example, salmon is delicious, but I don't hear anybody complaining about how they are "addicted" to it.

Natural foods are either high in carbohydrates (plant foods like potatoes and rice) or fat (animal foods like eggs, meat, and butter), but not in both. Ultra-processed foods often combine carbohydrates and fats to produce a peak in the "bliss point," the point where improved texture and mouthfeel create maximum pleasure. Functional MRI studies of the brain show that combining carbs with fat produces "supra-additive effects," meaning that the rewarding effect is more than the sum of either alone. The combination of carbs + fat is preferred far more than either alone.[24] Interesting.

This finding jibes with what common sense tells us. Baked potato chips (refined carbs) taste pretty so-so. Deep-fried potato chips (refined carbs + fats) are highly addictive. Low-fat rice cakes (refined carbs) are kind of meh. Ice cream (refined carbs + fats) can be addictive.

Many addictive substances contain flavor enhancers. Virtually nobody drinks purified 100 percent alcohol. Instead, it is commonly flavored, whether by aging in a barrel or adding sugars or other fruit flavors. Similarly, pure starch (boiled turnip) or pure fat (olive oil) is not particularly appetizing by itself, but add a little flavor and the result is transformative. Both salt and non-nutritive sweeteners may play a role in adding flavor. The following are the most common addictive foods[25]:

- Pizza
- Chocolate
- Chips
- Cookies
- Ice cream
- French fries
- Cheeseburgers
- Soda drinks (not diet)

This is a great list of foods to avoid for weight loss. The following are the least addictive foods:

- Cucumbers
- Carrots
- Beans (no sauce)
- Apples
- Brown rice
- Broccoli
- Bananas
- Salmon

131

Notably, low-calorie sweeteners also may activate some of the rewarding neurotransmitters, leading to addiction. Even though the sweeteners contain no calories, that doesn't mean they have no effect on eating behavior.[26] It's the hunger, not the calories, that count. When was the last time a friend told you: "I just switched to diet soda and lost 20 pounds"? Never? Yeah, me too. But many patients have told me that when they cut out the diet drinks, they effortlessly lost weight. The sweeteners can play an enabling role in creating a food addiction.

TREATING FOOD CRAVINGS AND FOOD ADDICTION

RECOGNIZING AN ADDICTION is the first step to treatment. The hallmark of any addiction is that you cannot stop doing a behavior (smoking, illicit drugs, eating) even though you recognize its destructive potential. These are some classic signs of food addiction:

- Feeling helpless or unable to stop eating
- Feeling out of control of one's own eating
- Eating past the point of comfort, but still unable to stop eating, and doing it again
- Eating more than intended, but still being unable to stop, and doing it again
- Feeling guilty about eating, but still being unable to stop, and doing it again
- Feeling an irresistible urge to eat even though you are full/not hungry
- Often hiding eating behavior, such as eating alone or very quickly
- Feeling guilt, shame, depression, or disgust after eating
- Trying unsuccessfully many times to quit disordered eating
- Making excuses—"It's just the one time" or "It's my spouse's fault"— to cover up disordered eating

132

Food addiction is a chronic condition. You might feel an overwhelming or uncontrollable desire to eat, whether you are hungry or not. A food craving is less severe and more common than addiction, occurring in an estimated 58 to 97 percent of people. A craving might feel like a strong urge for a particular food, by association with a smell or emotion or situation, or for no apparent reason. Eating even a little of the foods you crave can ignite an intense urge to eat more, which can lead to overeating and, over time, to addiction.

The best way to treat food addictions and cravings is with abstinence.[27] Do you tell a person with alcohol addiction to "just drink less" or a heroin user to "just use drugs less"? If you are addicted to UPFs, then the treatment strategy of moderation makes no sense.

Severe restrictions on eating the foods you crave can help break the habit and the conditioned response that follows. For example, fasting can abolish all cravings in response to the sight of food.[28] At the very least, extreme reduction is better than moderation.[29] In the case of alcohol and heroin, we understand just how profoundly idiotic that advice of moderation is. But in the case of food addiction, we think moderation is the height of scientific proof and inevitability. "Everything in moderation is fine," people say, smug in their ignorance of food addiction.

Critics argue that you cannot entirely abstain from food, but this argument misses the point. A person with a food addiction does not need to abstain from *all* foods, just those foods that are addictive, usually UPFs. A person addicted to drinking alcohol does not need to abstain from drinking green tea. A person addicted to refined carbohydrates does not need to abstain from eating eggs.

Unfortunately, food addictions are heavily stigmatized. If you are unable to resist the call of the donut, then many people consider it your fault, a lack of willpower or some other character defect. This belief makes getting help for food addiction that much harder. Both food and drugs are powerful rewards for human behavior, which, under the appropriate conditions, can overwhelm the body's homeostatic mechanism.

133

Treating an addiction is complex, requiring strategies like abstinence, cognitive behavioral therapy, peer group support (like Alcoholics Anonymous), positive psychology, and counseling. Taxing UPFs, limiting their availability to minors, and policy measures such as bans on advertising to children (as in tobacco) are other strategies. People need help to fight their addiction and to understand that an addiction is not a lack of willpower. People with food addiction do *not* need useless admonitions about why obesity or eating junk food is bad for them.

The sight, smell, or anticipation of an addictive substance can be enough to trigger longing and a rise in dopamine. This is why tobacco advertising is largely banned in North America, and we've been rewarded with a long steady decline in smoking. If you have a food addiction, you may need to change your behaviors or your environment. You might, for example, switch to streaming television to avoid the constant advertisements for UPFs on cable channels. Or you might change your social networks, just as smokers may need to find new non-smoking friends to avoid temptation and relapse.

Importantly, the first scientific trials published on treating food addictions have shown substantial promise. A low-carbohydrate, real food diet combined with online group counseling showed "significant, sustained improvement in ultra-processed food addiction symptoms and mental well-being."[30] Hopefully, increased recognition of food addiction can lead to better treatments and less stigma.

> **Tip #31:** Learn to recognize signs of food addiction,
> abstain from ultra-processed foods, and seek support.

8

MANAGING
EMOTIONAL EATING

ROXANE GAY, the *New York Times* bestselling author, weighed 577 pounds (261 kg) at her heaviest. In her brutally honest memoir entitled *Hunger: A Memoir of (My) Body*,[1] she explains that the word "obesity" "is an unpleasant word from the Latin 'obesus' meaning 'having eaten until fat,' which is, in a literal sense, fair enough." The real question is not *whether* she ate until fat, but *why*? Upon reflection, Gay believes that her early childhood sexual trauma precipitated her disordered relationship with food. Gay writes: "The past is written on my body. I carry it every single day. The past sometimes feels like it might kill me. It is a very heavy burden."

Gay understood the essence of the problem. Her memoir is not titled "Calories" or "Willpower" but, tellingly, "Hunger." The problem is not that Gay didn't know the health risks of obesity. The problem is not the lack of macronutrients, like protein. The problem is not the lack of vitamins or supplements. The problem is not the lack of exercise. The problem is the *hunger*.

We eat because we are hungry. The weight gain is only a symptom of the underlying problem: hunger. That's why the weight-loss advice to just Eat Less is futile. While technically correct, this sound-bite advice is useless in the real world, and highly derogatory besides. To solve a problem, you must treat the root cause, not the symptom.

There are many different types of hunger. Gay writes: "Hunger is in the mind and the body and the heart and the soul." That's exactly right. What we normally think of as hunger is properly called homeostatic hunger, the physiological impulse to eat that is triggered by hunger and satiety mechanisms to maintain homeostasis? But the physiology is only half the story, and in many cases, not even half. We eat for so many reasons other than homeostatic hunger. If Gay were eating to create a sense of mental safety, then no amount of well-meaning but senseless advice to "Eat Less" to improve her physical health will help.

The word "hedonic" means "relating to pleasure," and hedonic hunger refers to food intake driven by reasons other than metabolic necessity, including the rewarding and motivational aspects of eating. We eat not only because we are physically hungry or nutrient deficient, but also simply because we want to. It's pleasurable. Eating makes us feel good. You don't eat dessert because you are hungry, but you eat it nonetheless. Why? So many reasons.

- It is delicious.
- You feel compelled to eat (food addiction/addiction transfer).
- It makes you feel better (comfort food).
- You feel lonely sad/angry/depressed (emotional eating).
- You are bored.
- It's a habit.
- Everybody else is eating.

136   Can we please, please stop pretending that overeating is simply a lack of willpower or knowledge, and that the solution is "energy balance"? Alcoholism is not an "alcohol balance" problem. Heroin addiction is not a "heroin balance" problem. The sinking of the *Titanic* is not an "iceberg balance" problem.

Social and psychological factors can easily overwhelm homeostatic signals. If food is satisfying a deep-rooted psychological hunger, then restricting food—whether with dieting, diet drugs, or bariatric surgery— does not fill that emotional hunger. Restricting food may work temporarily, but it is a Band-Aid on a bullet wound.

WHAT IS EMOTIONAL EATING?

EMOTIONAL EATING IS the tendency to eat to soothe or suppress negative emotions or enhance positive emotions, and it is a vastly underappreciated factor in weight gain. Fifty-eight percent of patients seeking help from obesity medicine specialists report issues with emotional eating, and women may be particularly affected.[3] Interestingly, children are rarely affected by emotional eating,[4] and usually respond to negative emotions by eating less. This behavior changes during adolescence, when overeating becomes the dominant response.[5]

For emotional eaters, food is a coping mechanism to deal with low mood, anxiety, stress, loneliness, sadness, fear, or fatigue. Why? Because food provides comfort. Food gives pleasure in a day devoid of it. Food often becomes the highlight of the day.

The most common emotions that trigger eating are depressive ones, including sadness, loneliness, and boredom. Anxiety (worry, confusion, nervousness) and anger (guilt, resentment, jealousy) are also prominent emotions for emotional eating, although less so compared to depression. The dopamine and serotonin neurotransmitters are believed to be largely responsible, and perhaps not coincidentally are also highly linked to depressive symptoms.

Eating can also be a way to celebrate. To mark special occasions, events, and holidays, we use food to boost our good mood so that our celebration will be the best day of the year. We eat when watching a movie or a major sports event, to enhance our enjoyment (or because we are bored). We eat to reward ourselves for completing a task or reaching a goal. We all know it happens. We've all done it. So why pretend this eating doesn't matter?

137

Eating to feel pleasure

Eating food gives us pleasure because it releases dopamine in the reward centers of the brain, the nucleus accumbens. Insulin amplifies this dopamine release. Animal studies show a 20 to 55 percent increase in dopamine release in response to higher insulin levels.[6] Originally, this dopamine reward would have ensured our survival, driving us to find and eat food even when it was scarce. But all foods are different. Just as some foods are more fattening than others, some foods are more rewarding, or comforting, than others.

What makes a great comfort food? A food that is easy to eat and quickly absorbed to deliver a quick "hit." A food with a high level of refined carbohydrates to maximize insulin and dopamine release. A food with low satiety so you can keep eating it for its dopamine buzz without getting full. A food that is easy to eat and optimized for flavor and mouthfeel, so you feel good physically and emotionally when you eat it.

Hello, ultra-processed foods.

Eating to relieve sadness or pain

When people are sad and need comfort, they reach for "comfort" foods, like mac 'n' cheese, cookies, ice cream, sugary snacks, french fries, potato chips, or mashed potatoes. Why?

Food is a way to self-medicate with a dopamine hit. It makes you feel better, albeit only temporarily. Wanting to feel better is understandable and rational behavior. Yet UPFs amp up the reward system, sometimes to the point of addiction. With their combination of convenience, soft texture, high dose of carbohydrates, rapid digestion and absorption, and poor satiety, UPFs are perfectly engineered to provide a massive glucose and insulin high to fire up your dopamine.

Natural foods don't lend themselves to emotional eating. Although a piece of salmon or eggplant is delicious, it doesn't cause the massive spike of glucose, insulin, and dopamine that UPFs do. You don't drown your sorrows in eggplant. I love eggplant, but it's definitely not a comfort food.

138

The mental relief brought on by UPFs doesn't last. The dopamine hit is fleeting, so you need to keep eating. Viewed this way, overeating dopamine-spiking UPFs is a logical and rational response to emotional hunger. But this chronic insulin stimulation leads to weight gain over time, and emotional eaters often feel they are losing control. When people realize how much weight they've gained and how difficult it is to stop eating comfort foods, they often feel guilt and shame, which only feeds the cycle of emotional eating and keeps it going.

Emotional eating is a big problem. Over half of all people with excess weight and obesity overeat in response to negative emotions.[7] In young women, higher body mass index is linked to higher rates of emotional eating.[8] In any given month, an estimated 38 percent of adults worldwide have engaged in emotional eating, and almost half engage in it weekly.[9]

Up to 50 percent of patients trying to lose weight have depression. The prevalence of depression in mild obesity is 11.4 percent, and that percentage increases as obesity increases.[10] Obesity can cause depression, but depression can also cause obesity, so it's often hard to know which is the chicken and which is the egg. An obese person has a 55 percent increased risk of being depressed. A person with depression has a 58 percent chance of becoming obese.[11]

The point is clear. It is impossible to separate the problems of obesity and mental health. Emotional hunger (loneliness, sadness, anxiety) drives us to look for the dopamine hit that comes from eating UPFs. Dieting or telling people to eat fewer calories will just produce feelings of deprivation, because the emotional hunger is not being satisfied. This deprivation mindset will doom any long-term diet.

What are the signs of emotional eating?

- You can't control your eating but you don't know why.
- You have a strong urge to eat whenever you feel strong emotions.
- You have an irresistible urge to eat even though you're not hungry.
- You find food calming.

If emotional eating is the problem, then the first step is to identify it. Then, dealing with the underlying emotional issue through counseling, therapy, meditation, and peer support is the treatment of choice.

Distracted or mindless eating

Emotional eating and distracted, or mindless, eating are linked through their shared roots in disrupted self-regulation and coping mechanisms. Both behaviors bypass mindful eating, and thus often feed into each other. Emotional eating is focused on seeking comfort from food. But sometimes we eat not because we are hungry or to make us feel better but just because we're not paying attention and the food is there.

For example, we eat while driving, watching television or a movie, having a meeting, or playing computer games. When we eat mindlessly, we may not notice what or how much we are eating. We may not even know if we are hungry or full.

Changes in social and societal norms have allowed distracted and mindless eating to rise. In the 1960s and 1970s in North America, you ate only at certain times and in certain places. You ate breakfast, lunch, and dinner. And that was all. No snacks, no coffee breaks. You ate in the kitchen, dining room, or cafeteria. No eating in your bedroom or the living room. No eating in front of the TV or at your desk. And no eating in meetings.

Today, we can eat whenever and wherever we want. With few rules about where we cannot eat, we are more at risk of mindless eating. The most common form of distracted eating is while watching TV (21.7%), but eating while online or while driving is also common. In the workplace, we hold "lunch meetings" to multitask and save time. We even walk down the street talking on our cell phones and wolfing down our food on the way to our next meeting. In one study, only 18.4 percent of people surveyed reported no distractions while eating. The consequences of mindless and distracted eating are predictable: increased body weight.[12]

> **Tip #32:** Avoid distracted eating.
> Eat only at a table in a designated place—kitchen,
> dining room—and turn off or put away tech devices.

Satiety requires attention and memory. But when we eat automatically out of habit, we are eating without full conscious awareness. And if you don't pay attention to your food, you won't notice that you're full.[13] If you don't pay attention to your food, you don't taste it and therefore you don't remember it. Then, not remembering you ate it, you'll get hungry again much sooner.[14]

When patients with amnesia who have just eaten a full meal are immediately offered more food, they eat almost a whole second meal. They "forget" to be full, so they eat again, as their hunger increases to match.[15] In other cases, some patients with amnesia rarely reported being hungry—almost as if they "forgot" to be hungry. What that finding suggests is that satiety may require some higher cognitive function to remember that we are full, to provide context to our situation.

Snacking is a common form of distracted, mindless eating. The food we eat mid-morning or mid-afternoon with coffee or during a break is not necessary. We often eat these snacks out of boredom, but these pastries or chocolate bars or potato chips or carrot sticks still count toward our weight gain. Eating while multitasking is also mindless eating.

To make food memorable, season it. Cook with herbs and spices, which naturally add flavor. Be bold with chilies and ingredients like anchovies and Parmesan cheese, which add umami. To pay more attention to your food, cultivate a mindful eating practice (page 144).

> **Tip #33:** Enhance your memory of food by choosing
> highly seasoned, spicy, and high-umami foods.

Once you've recognized that you are using food as an emotional support, you can look for alternative coping strategies that are healthier, including goal setting, positive mindset, positive self-talk, journaling, and cognitive behavioral therapy. The full scope of dealing with the negative emotions that underlie emotional eating is far beyond this book. However, mindful eating can provide a stable foundation for dealing with emotional hunger and distracted eating. Learning to manage the stress that leads to emotional eating, by regulating the vagus nerve, is another strategy you can try.

PRACTICING MINDFUL EATING

MINDFULNESS-BASED TREATMENTS ARE highly effective for weight loss, cost nothing, and produce lasting results. Mindful eating is to be aware of what, how much, and why we are eating. Most importantly, mindful eating teaches awareness and acceptance.

Many of us are consciously aware of homeostatic hunger. We feel hunger pangs and we eat. We are less consciously aware of the associated pleasure of eating. Both are important: we need to be aware of both what and why we are eating. We don't necessarily need to change the reason, but we need to acknowledge and accept it.

Mindfulness teaches you to accept your food choices and the reasons for eating those foods. You cultivate "inner wisdom," the ability to make decisions to suit complex situations. That's very different from a "dieting mindset," which imposes set rules regardless of circumstance. Mindfulness means becoming aware of hunger (all kinds), eating triggers, emotions, and thoughts. This awareness is the first step toward potentially healthier ways of coping. That is, rather than focusing on foods, diets, or nutrients as the dieting mindset does, mindfulness targets the underlying attentional or emotional stimulus to eat. Mindful eating is a treatment for hedonic hunger, not homeostatic hunger.

Mindful eating might seem cumbersome at first. With practice, it becomes second nature and only takes a few extra minutes. It's a treatment that demands attention, not time. Perhaps that is why the benefits of mindful eating for weight loss increase rather than fade over time. Mindfulness becomes easier the more you practice it.

A review of fifteen studies involving 560 people found that the average weight loss after using a mindfulness-based treatment was 4.2 kg (9.3 pounds). More stunning is that average weight loss increased over the six-month follow-up period to 9.2 kg (20 pounds)![16] Another meta-analysis of studies estimated that mindful eating reduces weight by 6.8 pounds (3.1 kg) on average and 7.5 pounds (3.4 kg) at follow-up.[17]

Hara hachi bu: Mantras for mindfulness

Using a short, simple mantra is a very powerful psychological technique that serves as a timely reminder to eat mindfully. The Japanese phrase "hara hachi bu" means roughly "Eat until you are 80 percent full." This phrase is believed to have originated with the philosopher Ekiken Kaibara in the 1713 book *Yojokun: Life Lessons From a Samurai*. And it is still in use today. When doing research in Okinawa, Japan, for his book about people who live measurably longer and healthier lives, Dan Buettner, author of *The Blue Zones: Secrets for Living Longer*, recalls older residents murmuring "hara hachi bu" before each meal. In Western culture, saying a prayer of gratitude or a blessing before a meal serves the same purpose. It is a reminder to give gratitude and therefore to eat mindfully.

The purpose of hara hachi bu, a prayer, or any other statement of intention is to eat mindfully, not necessarily to eat less. After all, how can you eat until you are 80 percent full unless you pay close attention? And how can you pay attention unless you also slow down your eating? This advice is especially great since it takes time for satiety signals to reach the brain. If you eat quickly and until you are completely stuffed, then you will find yourself way too full, to the point of being sick. Yet you won't realize it until you have already eaten well past the point of satisfying your hunger.

How to eat mindfully

Allow time and be intentional about what you're eating.

Before you eat

1. Take three deep breaths. Look around. Who are you eating with? Where are you? Consider your surroundings.
2. Recite a mantra such as hara hachi bu or other words of your choosing to remind yourself to eat mindfully. You can murmur this mantra under your breath, if necessary.

As you are eating

3. Consider why you are eating. Emotional comfort? Boredom? Routine?
4. Consider how hungry you really are.
5. Consider each piece of food. Is it ultra-processed? Is it highly refined? Is it full of sugar? You can still eat it, but just admit it. That's the point of mindfulness. You aren't making a judgment, just acknowledging a fact to make a conscious decision to eat or not eat.
6. Use all your senses. Consider how the food looks, smells, tastes, feels, and sounds. Enjoy it. Food is meant to be savored. Appreciate it.
7. Take one bite of food, chew thoroughly, and eat slowly. Put down your utensil every few bites to allow you to savor your food and enjoy your company.
8. After each mouthful, take a few seconds to consider how you feel before picking up your utensils again. Make a conscious decision to eat or stop and understand why. Listen to your stomach, not your plate.
9. Focus on how you feel—both physically and emotionally. How are those sensations changing? Do you feel yourself getting full? Are you satisfied? Take your time, stay present, and don't rush the experience.

After you finish eating

10. Give gratitude for being here in this time and place and enjoying the food.
11. Keep talking with your dining companions. Enjoy their company.

12. Reflect on your meal. Did you manage to eat mindfully? Could you have done anything differently? Did you cope with emotional hunger?
13. Make a point to remember what you just ate.
14. Write down what you ate and your thoughts while eating. Food journaling is a powerful tool for self-discovery.

Mindful eating is a tool to stay present in the moment, savoring and giving gratitude for food, and understanding the reasons why you are eating what you are eating. It is not a way to deprive yourself. It is not about being perfect. You might still eat UPFs or eat for emotional hunger, but at least you'll know why. You are practicing self-acceptance, not willpower and powering through. So remember to be gentle with yourself. Acknowledge when you eat with awareness. And when you don't, renew your intention to try again at the next meal.

Tip #34: Cultivate a mindful eating practice
(and keep a food journal).

LEARNING TO CALM YOUR VAGUS NERVE

THE VAGUS NERVE is the longest nerve in the body, and it is part of the parasympathetic nervous system (PNS) that governs calmness, relaxation, digestion, mood, and even inflammation. Dr. Vernon B. Williams, a sports neurologist at Cedars-Sinai hospital writes: "It turns out that many of the activities that we associate with calmness—things like deep breathing, meditation, massage, and even the experience of awe—effect changes in the brain, in part, through increasing vagus nerve activity."[18] You can't always control the things that cause you stress, but you can control your body's reaction to that stress. Using some simple relaxation techniques can help to slow your heart rate and soothe emotional hunger.

Each of these topics is far beyond our scope here. Indeed, entire books have been written about each of these subjects. My goal is only to point you in the right direction.

145

1. **Regular deep breathing.** Use this technique to relax the mind and stimulate the parasympathetic nervous system. The simplest method is to breathe in slowly, smoothly, and without force through your nose for four seconds. Immediately breathe out for four to six seconds without pausing.

   A slightly more advanced variation is box breathing. Breathe in for four seconds, hold your breath for four seconds, breathe out for four seconds, and hold your breath for four seconds.

2. **Meditation.** Use this technique to calm your mind by bringing your attention to a specific action, object, thought, or activity. Closely observe your breath, slowly repeat a mantra, or look at the details in a visual image.

3. **Stretching/yoga.** Slowing down and releasing tension in your body by stretching can help your mind relax too. Try gentle forms of yoga or lengthening poses in a cool, quiet space.

4. **Exercise/movement.** Moving your body brings oxygen to the brain, which improves your mood. Choose the exercise and the pace that's right for you, whether it's walking, swimming, bicycling, or a game of tennis with friends.

5. **Cold exposure.** Start by turning the water to "cold" for the last ten seconds of your shower. Gradually build up to thirty seconds of cold water. If you're brave, try immersing your body completely in a cold bath or a lake. Exposure to cold water also releases endorphins and improves mood.

6. **Laugh, even if you don't feel like it.** The simple act of smiling or laughing improves your mood. It's almost like your brain notices you laughing and then figures, "We must be in a good mood."

7. **Grounding.** Walk in your bare feet on the beach, on your lawn, or just in the dirt. Feel your connection to the earth. This practice, called grounding or earthing, is very relaxing and feels surprisingly good.[19]

8. **Nature walking/forest bathing/hiking.** Spending time in nature relaxes the body and reduces stress.

9. **Massage/acupuncture.** Gentle to moderate pressure or stimulation, particularly in the neck, shoulders, and feet, can activate the PNS and bring calm to your body and mind.

All these treatments have potentially large benefits and almost no risk of harm. As always, when you're feeling emotional, look for support from your peers—family, friends, neighbors, acquaintances from church or work, and so on. Spending time with people you like can help you relax and improve your mood.

> **Tip #35:** Relax your body to activate the vagus nerve
> and reduce stress-related eating.

ANTICIPATING LIFE CHANGES

SOME EXPERIENCES CAN be especially stressful and lead to emotional eating, such as going to college, getting married, and entering menopause. At these times, using your mindful eating and relaxation strategies can really help.

The transition from high school to college often is accompanied by weight gain. This occurrence is so well known that it is sometimes nicknamed the Freshman 15, for the expected weight gain of 6.8 kg (15 pounds).[20] The college diet is famously full of alcohol, junk food, and sugar, along with lifestyle changes like increased stress and poor sleeping habits.

In the U.S., marriage is associated with weight gain for men, but not for women. The reasons are not obvious, since most men's diet doesn't change much.[21] If anything, I would expect the quality of the diet to improve, given the notoriously bad eating habit of bachelors. It is possible that the increased stress of child-rearing and loss of sleep may play a role in developing a Dad bod.

Women who menstruate experience fluctuations in food intake through their cycle. During the first half of the cycle, the follicular phase, estrogen is building up and peaks at ovulation. This is accompanied by decreased food intake. After ovulation, progesterone increases, and with it, hunger, which causes women to eat more. Fasting is often easier in the follicular phase due to the decreased hunger. Perimenopause, however, changes those patterns. The perimenopausal period is often accompanied by weight gain, due to the decreased estrogen. In one study, women gained an average of 2.25 kg (5 pounds) over a three-year period during perimenopause. For many women, the stress of life changes around this time can also lead to emotional eating.[22]

Both homeostatic hunger and hedonic hunger are important aspects of eating behavior that can, if dysfunctional, lead to weight gain. But together, they still do not fully describe what drives us to eat and overeat because they do not account for the social, learned, and associative aspects of food, which we call conditioned hunger. Part 3 helps us to understand this third type of hunger.

GLORIA

Gloria was addicted to food. For most of her life, she'd found temptation everywhere, and once she started eating, she found it very hard to stop. To compensate, she tried all the fad and calorie-reduction diets. Predictably, none of them brought long-term success. Eight years ago, she learned about fasting.

"Intermittent fasting has been a game-changer because it helps to break all those bad habits," says Gloria. It is "realistic magic." Today she's perimenopausal, and instead of gaining weight as many women do, she's lost weight. Fasting has also helped resolve the joint pain that began in her hands about a year ago.

She follows three commandments: follow time-restricted eating to break the cycle of eating constantly, know how and when to keep insulin levels under control, and "get back on the horse when you fall off." Gloria has seen many health benefits and is committed to making these commandments a lifelong practice.

ANASTASIA

Anastasia was forty when she was diagnosed with type 2 diabetes and was prescribed multiple medications. She immediately switched to a vegan diet, yet her weight and her insulin prescription continued to climb. By age forty-six, she had reached 372 pounds (168 kg), she was using over 200 units of insulin daily, and her legs were so swollen she could barely walk. How was that possible? After all, she was taking her medications. She was eating a vegan diet. She was eating six times a day. And she was measuring and weighing all her food! Despite following all her doctor's recommendations, she felt hopeless.

Over the previous years, Anastasia had divorced, and she was caring for her mother with late-stage breast cancer while working full-time. Why was she eating? Stress! Once she realized that she was eating emotionally, she was able to get support and we developed a plan.

Although she'd been eating a vegan diet, it was full of refined carbs and fake meat. She switched to natural foods and began to eat salads, meat, eggs, and dairy instead. She incorporated fasting—starting gently and building up. As she did, her blood sugar came down and her meds were carefully adjusted as she healed. The swelling in her legs disappeared in less than two weeks! And she was able to stop taking all the insulin and most of the other medications within a month.

Anastasia lost over 150 pounds (68 kg) and has kept it off for more than two years. Best of all, she's active, energetic, and better able to handle stress without eating.

LEE

As a teenager, Lee developed a taste for vending-machine snacks—processed foods loaded with fat and sugar. She was so addicted to refined carbohydrates that she couldn't stop eating for even twelve hours, including sleep time! She used to wake at 3 a.m. to raid the refrigerator, and during the day she couldn't go four hours without a carb fix. For decades, Lee's eating followed a similar pattern: watching the scale creep steadily upward then dieting obsessively to try to bring it back down. She had yo-yoed through every popular diet, eventually reaching her heaviest weight of 350 pounds (159 kg).

Finally recognizing the problem, she began to fast and was gradually able to go without eating for sixteen to eighteen hours. In four and a half months, she lost more than 50 pounds (23 kg), simply by cutting out snacks between meals, late-night eating, and processed carbohydrates. On that foundation, she added longer fasts and has now lost 160 pounds (73 kg) total. She's also reversed her type 2 diabetes and high blood pressure; reduced her migraines, brain fog, allergies, skin problems, and joint pain; and improved her overall mood.

Has she slipped? Yes, occasionally. When her aunt passed away a couple of years ago, she began to stress-eat late at night and the pounds crept back. But being mindful has allowed her to recognize the issue, be gentle with herself, and recommit to her own health—and to helping others. At age seventy, she's become a lifestyle coach, sharing her newfound knowledge with others.

PART
THREE

Conditioned Hunger

| 9 |

LIVING IN AN OBESOGENIC ENVIRONMENT

THE COMMON NARRATIVE of obesity in America says that the problem lies with the individual, that obesity is fundamentally an individual's lack of willpower. Even a cursory look at the scientific evidence shows that this belief is false. Think about it this way. Suppose that in a classroom of a hundred children, one child fails. Perhaps the child is at fault. They didn't study. They watched too much TV or played too many video games instead of doing their schoolwork. But what if seventy children fail? The problem is more likely a systemic factor: the school curriculum or the teacher's methods. Berating the children and haranguing them to Play Less, Study More won't work, because the children aren't the problem. Instead, it is far more useful to assess the school, the teacher, and the learning environment.

In the U.S., about 70 percent of adults have a body mass index in the overweight or obese range. Is this an individual problem, or a systemic one? Instead of berating and haranguing people to Eat Less, Move More, we should focus on the environment—societal and social—that has led to the obesity epidemic. Why do people who move to the U.S. often get fat? The dominant factors, which I feel are massively underappreciated, are the macro-environment (society, country, region) that surrounds us and the micro-environment that we surround ourselves with (our friends, family, and households). These external factors influence our individual beliefs and values through behavioral processes like conditioning and social modeling. Maintaining a healthy weight in an external environment that promotes excessive weight gain—an obesogenic environment—is like trying to stay afloat in a tsunami.

WHERE YOU LIVE AFFECTS YOUR WEIGHT

UNTIL THE 1970S, Americans enjoyed low rates of obesity without effort or willpower. Today, the number of Americans with obesity has exploded. As of 2024, a full 74 percent of Americans were considered overweight or obese, and the number is projected to rise to more than 80 percent by 2050.[1] What changed? Not the individual. Human nature has not changed much in the last fifty years. What has changed dramatically is the society we live in and its food environment and social norms. Society provides the structural framework and systems that shape our lives. When government policies, cultural norms, and the places we live in encourage obesity, then we are likely to gain weight.

Obesity rates in the U.S. are much higher than in many other countries around the world. Americans eat 3868 calories per day, putting them second on the list of the world's biggest eaters.[2] In contrast, the average Japanese person eats 2705 calories per day, ranking that country at #125 on the list. The critical question we need to answer is not *whether* Americans eat more than Japanese people but *why*. Americans don't individually *choose* to eat more so that they can gain a lot of unwelcome body fat. Obviously, obesity is a systemic issue that reflects a country's social and cultural influence on our diet.

The truth is this. When you live (1970s versus 2020s) and where you live (U.S. versus Japan) matters more than who you are. Is weight gain nature (genetics) or nurture (environment)? Science reveals very clearly that nurture plays the bigger role in obesity. What this information tells us is that while each of us makes individual decisions about what we eat and when, as a society we will not achieve lasting weight loss until we shift our food environment and our thinking. The easiest way to understand the relative contributions of the individual versus the society is to study people who move from one place to another—immigrants.

People who immigrate to the U.S. are typically thin. After they live in the U.S. for a while, most get fat. It doesn't matter much whether they come from poor nations or rich nations. It doesn't matter much whether they are Black, white, Latino, or Asian. People from every immigrant group in the world get fat when they move to the U.S. One study found that immigrants who had lived in the U.S. for less than a year had a mind-bogglingly low 8 percent rate of obesity. By the time these immigrants had lived for fifteen years in the U.S., 57 percent were overweight or obese, which is similar to the percentage for people born in the U.S.[3]

Consider a person who moves from Japan to the U.S. Both Japan and the U.S. are wealthy, modern nations. The first generation of immigrants who were born and raised in Japan but moved to the U.S. (Issei) had a rate of overweight or obesity of 25.2 percent. By the second generation, people of Japanese descent who were born and raised in the U.S. (Nisei), that rate of overweight or obesity had ballooned to 43.6 percent.[4] The cause of the weight gain wasn't their genetics. It was the environment: societal and cultural norms which the immigrants were assimilating. Living in an obesogenic environment, these people of Japanese descent stood no chance.

Even by 1991, twenty-five years after the first arrivals in the study, the prevalence of obesity of all Japanese people living in California was *quadruple* the rate of a Japanese person living in Japan.[5] Tellingly, the longer a person had lived in the U.S., the fatter they were. Living in Japan rather than in the U.S. automatically makes you less likely to be overweight.

Within the U.S., some regions are more obesogenic than others. For example, the southeastern U.S. is associated with very high levels of obesity, high blood pressure, heart disease, stroke, and type 2 diabetes. The "Southern diet" is not particularly high in calories (about 2000 per day) or carbohydrates (50 percent carbohydrates, 35 percent fat), so why is it so unhealthy? The Southern diet is dominated by UPFs; it is high in fried foods, added fats (mostly vegetable oils), processed meats, white bread, and sugar-sweetened beverages. When the eating environment is dominated by ultra-processed carbs fried in ultra-processed vegetable oil with ultra-processed meats (proteins) along with lots of sugary drinks, obesity is almost unavoidable.[6]

California cuisine, on the other hand, emphasizes fresh, local, and seasonal foods rather than UPFs. Not coincidentally, obesity rates are relatively low in California, at 27.7 percent, and relatively high in the American South (Mississippi), at 40.1 percent.[7]

> **Tip #36:** Remember that where you live has powerful effects on your personal health, including body weight.

Social modeling, or how our environment shapes us through observation and imitation, is the key link between population-level influences and individual actions.

SOCIAL MODELING

WHAT DO YOU want to be when you grow up? As a child, I dreaded being asked that inane question that always seemed to be the first thing an adult wanted to know. Back in the day, popular answers included teacher, doctor, police officer, firefighter, and nurse. But times have changed. A 2022 survey found that a staggering 57 percent of young people (Generation Z) want to grow up to be... a social media influencer.[8] This finding illustrates the overwhelming importance of social influence and social modeling on our everyday lives—and yes, on eating behavior, too.

158   All of us learn by observing and copying others. This social modeling is an incredibly pervasive and powerful force in shaping behaviors. As children, we observe a role model, usually a parent or sibling, and mimic their behaviors, speech, and eating patterns. This modeling

provides us with a reference of what is normal and acceptable, and includes food choices, eating schedules, and size of meals. As we get older, we still gather these cues, though often from our friends or from influencers or celebrities we admire.

Eating, like drinking alcohol and smoking cigarettes, is heavily influenced by where we live because our environment determines the social norms—the range of behaviors that are considered socially and culturally acceptable. Social influence is automatic and unconscious, so people are usually unaware of just how much it can contribute to weight gain. For example, when families in the U.S. Army were assigned to a military base in a county with higher obesity rates, those families gained weight. For every 1 percent increase in the rate of obesity in the county they moved to, the teenagers in the family increased their risk of obesity by 5 percent.[9] If your best friend becomes obese, your own risk increases by a staggering *171 percent.* If your sibling becomes obese, your risk increases by 40 percent. Geographic distance is less important than social distance. The food environment and social norms that you share among your family and friends make a huge difference.[10]

If your best friend always eats salad instead of french fries, that food choice rubs off. If your best friend runs every day, that lifestyle choice rubs off. If your best friend eats junk food and snacks all day and night, that habit rubs off. Obesity spreads like contagion along social ties because behaviors rub off.

People eat more when others around them eat more, and less when others eat less. People eat more often if others around them eat more often. People eat the same kinds of foods as others around them are eating. The current North American dietary environment, compared to other countries and its own history, encourages people to:

1. **Eat more.** Portions in the United States are much larger than those in Japan or Europe, so it is socially acceptable and "normal" to eat more.
2. **Eat more often (and fast less often).** In the 1970s, most people ate three times per day: breakfast, lunch, and dinner. By 2004,

people were eating almost double that, at six times per day.[11] That's breakfast, snack, lunch, snack, dinner, and then before bed, you guessed it, another snack.

3. **Eat quickly and while doing other things.** Mindless and distracted eating is socially acceptable and common.

4. **Eat more ultra-processed foods.** UPFs dominate the diets of the U.S. and U.K., but less so in Japan and Italy (Figure 9.1).[12]

Figure 9.1. People in the U.S. and the U.K. eat a much higher percentage of ultra-processed foods of the total calories they consume than all other countries

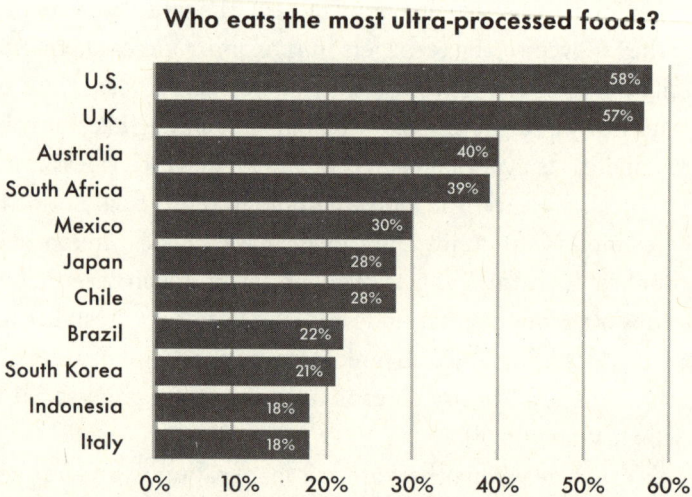

Who eats the most ultra-processed foods?

Country	Percentage
U.S.	58%
U.K.	57%
Australia	40%
South Africa	39%
Mexico	30%
Japan	28%
Chile	28%
Brazil	22%
South Korea	21%
Indonesia	18%
Italy	18%

That is a surefire recipe for an epidemic of obesity. The "experts" obsess about individual responsibility, but by far the biggest influences on eating behavior are the macro- and micro-environments that surround us.

> **Tip #37:** Observe how the social and cultural norms of the people around you influence your eating behavior.

WHAT MAKES SOME PLACES SO PRONE TO OBESITY?

THE U.S. HAS higher levels of obesity than many other countries. The American South has higher levels of obesity than other parts of the U.S. Why are some places so obesogenic? Many factors come into play:

- The ubiquity of ultra-processed foods (24/7 coffee shops, fast-food restaurants, convenience stores, drive-thrus, food delivery services)
- The endless choice of ultra-processed and fast foods (burgers, pizza and other Italian food, Chinese food, Thai food, Japanese food, and so on)
- The low cost of ultra-processed foods (due to agricultural subsidies and economies of scale when food is produced on industrial mega-farms)
- The constant marketing and advertising of ultra-processed foods
- A food culture that emphasizes quantity (all you can eat) over quality
- A built environment that promotes driving as opposed to walking or other active forms of transportation

All these factors apply around the world, but they are most obvious in the U.S. Ultra-processed foods dominate the American diet more than virtually any other country on earth. This list of factors is not exhaustive and serves only to illustrate that many factors beyond simple individual choice affect weight. However, let's look at a few of these factors in more detail.

The ubiquity of ultra-processed foods

Hunger increases when you think about food or when you see, smell, or anticipate food. The thought of fresh popcorn in the theater suddenly makes you hungry. Seeing a billboard or television advertisement for chips or ice cream makes you suddenly crave those foods. The smell of freshly baked cinnamon buns wafting through the mall suddenly makes you hungry when you weren't before. It's no accident that there are trays of tempting donuts whenever you buy a coffee. The French have a saying, "You eat first with your eyes," to describe the anticipation of eating.

Most of us are surrounded by food cues all the time, which means we are often thinking about food whether that thought is conscious or not. Sometimes the sight or smell of food nearby triggers our thinking about food. Sometimes the trigger is a memory—your grandma's freshly cooked dumplings, or your family's holiday turkey with all the trimmings. Either way, these thoughts activate sensory signals that anticipate food and trigger hunger. The body's physiological responses to these signals are called the cephalic phase responses (CPRs),[13] and they can determine whether and how much we eat.

CPRs prepare us for digestion. You start to salivate; your stomach starts growling as it starts moving; your pancreas starts secreting digestive enzymes. Importantly, from a weight standpoint, the hormones insulin and ghrelin are released, which together begin storing calories (as sugar and fat) and increasing hunger to feed this storage.

The ubiquity of easily available food can make CPRs a conditioned response to the thought, anticipation, sight, smell, taste, texture, and mouthfeel of food. Online food delivery services, fast food, quick casual, and regular restaurants are everywhere. Coffee shops sell coffee *and* a full array of tempting baked goods, including lunch items. Many gas stations sell you fuel for your car plus a whole array of snack foods at the till plus fast foods at an outlet inside. Hotels, office buildings, theaters, arenas, stadiums, community centers, and hospitals have multiple food sellers in the lobby and vending machines in the halls. Even your home office can cue your conditioned hunger if you work very close to your kitchen or *in* your kitchen. Everywhere you turn, there's food. Everywhere you turn, you are activating your CPRs.

To reduce hunger, reduce the mention and expectation of food. You can't always change your environment, but you can remove yourself from food, and you can remove food from your immediate living, working, and recreating spaces. Remove food from as many environments that you can control as possible—the car, the TV room, your workstation. Plan a route that doesn't go by your workplace cafeteria or the snack bar at the theater. Don't work in your kitchen or in coffee shops. Other steps might be to stream your TV shows rather than watching them on cable networks, to avoid food commercials. Try not to watch food shows. Avoid shopping in a mall, so you can skip the food court, the chocolate shops, and the specialty bakeries and bubble tea shops. When I order my coffee, I generally do it using an app on my phone, to avoid the temptation of seeing and smelling the donuts and cookies.

> **Tip #38:** Avoid or remove from your environment anything that will trigger thoughts of food.

The low cost of ultra-processed foods

Food availability is influenced heavily by price. If foods are cheaper, people will eat more of them and more often. Low-cost food is a significant reason why the U.S. is such a fattening society.

The U.S. government provides substantial agricultural subsidies, but these are not equally distributed. In 2024, corn growers received $3.2 billion and soybean farmers received close to $2 billion, while wheat subsidies ranked fourth (Figure 9.2[14]).[15] Subsidies often lead growers to overproduce these crops, which drives prices down. Food manufacturers use this river of cheap corn and wheat (highly refined carbohydrates) and soybean oil (highly refined oil) to produce UPFs, which they can sell for much cheaper than healthier natural foods like vegetables, which receive barely any subsidies.

Nutrition data bears out this fact. In the U.S., 56.2 percent of calories consumed are from the most subsidized foods (corn, soy, wheat, rice, sorghum, dairy, and livestock). That number rises to between 66 and 100 percent among those with less education, living in poverty, and less food secure.[16]

Globally, government subsidies for agriculture amount to approximately $600 billion a year.[17] In 2022, Dr. Máximo Torero Cullen, chief economist of the Food and Agriculture Organization of the United Nations, noted: "Rice, sugar and meat of various types are the foods most incentivized worldwide, while producers of fruits and vegetables are less supported overall, and even penalized in some low-income countries."[18] In other words, with agricultural subsidies, governments very often have different objectives than ensuring human health.

Figure 9.2. The U.S. government provided more than $5 billion in subsidies to corn and soybean growers in 2024

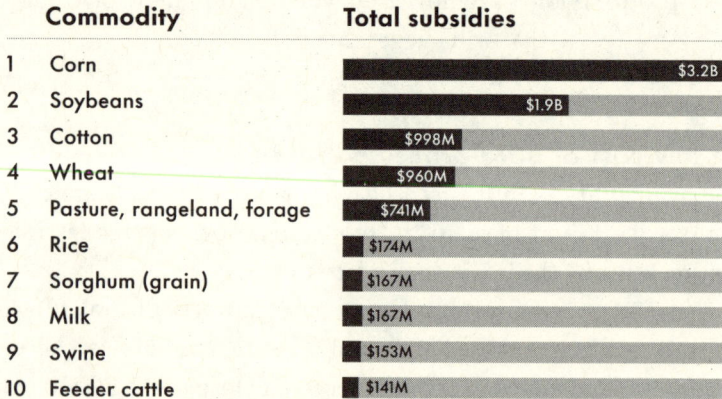

	Commodity	Total subsidies
1	Corn	$3.2B
2	Soybeans	$1.9B
3	Cotton	$998M
4	Wheat	$960M
5	Pasture, rangeland, forage	$741M
6	Rice	$174M
7	Sorghum (grain)	$167M
8	Milk	$167M
9	Swine	$153M
10	Feeder cattle	$141M

The constant marketing and advertising of ultra-processed foods

Companies spend billions every year on food and alcohol advertising in the U.S., much of which goes toward promoting fast food and UPFs. A large part of the advertising is TV ads, but spending on digital and social media advertising is rapidly increasing, as is food influencer marketing.[19] Advertising keeps reminding us of food hunger.

Generally, we can't change macro-environmental factors, but we can create a micro-environment (family, friends, personal habits) for positive change. The first step is to understand how we internalize these external cues to eat. Where we live determines our conditioned habits and social norms—the range of expectations and behaviors that are considered socially and culturally acceptable. Social influence, expectations, and conditioning are automatic and unconscious, so people are usually unaware of just how much they can contribute to weight gain.

| 10 |

RECOGNIZING
EATING AS A HABIT

A FEW YEARS AGO, I overheard a parent begging their child to please eat a few more bites of their hot dog before they could have ice cream. The child was putting up a huge fuss. I remember wondering, "Why force a child to eat junk food by bribing them with dessert? If they're not hungry, just don't feed them. Then everybody wins. The child doesn't eat food they don't want, and the parent knows the child is not eating so much junk food." The whole argument seemed rather silly to me, and so I reflected on the underlying issue.

Why do we eat? We like to think it's because we are hungry, but many times we eat simply out of habit. It's breakfast time, so we eat. It's lunchtime, so we eat. It's dinnertime so, you guessed it, we eat. This habitual eating does not happen naturally. Small children won't eat if they are not hungry, no matter what time it is. When they don't want to eat, we beg them to do so: "No dessert until you finish your dinner!" "You can't leave the table until you finish eating." "Don't leave food on your plate."

This constant chorus trains children to eat at specific times rather than listening to their body's natural hunger and satiety signals. Over time, eating becomes a habit—a learned behavior that becomes mostly involuntary. And habits are incredibly important because they form the baseline, or default setting, for what we do.

Society sets the tone for some of these habits, but we internalize and perpetuate them because of the people around us. We make our habits, and then our habits make us.

LEARNING BY ASSOCIATION: THE CONDITIONED RESPONSE

IN THE 1890S, famed Russian physiologist Ivan Pavlov was studying the process of digestion in dogs. Specifically, he was looking at the role of saliva in breaking down food. Every day, a technician brought food for the dogs, and the dogs would naturally salivate in response to the sight of that food. Soon, however, Pavlov noted astutely that the dogs began to salivate when they saw the technician, before the food was even brought out. The dogs had learned that seeing the technician meant food was coming, and they started to salivate in anticipation. Pavlov was one of the first people to describe the phenomenon now called classical conditioning.

Intrigued by the dogs' response, Pavlov next paired the ringing of a bell with the appearance of the food. The sound of a bell is a neutral stimulus, since dogs won't naturally salivate when they hear a bell. After repeatedly hearing the bell with the food, the dogs began to salivate when they heard the ringing, before any food was available. This response is known as a learned, or conditioned, response, and this experiment helped lay the foundations of modern behavioral psychology.

Why do we care? Because **hunger is also a conditioned response**. That is, much of our "hunger" is a learned behavior. Through repetition, we learn to associate certain external food cues with eating. Cues are triggers or reminders to engage in a habit. When we pair the cue with the many different motivations to eat (boredom, loneliness, food addictions, and so on), the urge to eat becomes irresistible. A two-year randomized controlled trial from Harvard University, published in

166

2017, confirmed that the more you eat certain foods, the more you will crave them, which supports the "conditioning model of food cravings."[1] Dr. David Kessler, author of *The End of Overeating*, has termed this phenomenon "conditioned hypereating."

Our internal cues are physical, like a growling tummy (homeostatic hunger), and emotional, like stress or depression (hedonic hunger). These cues come from inside our body. We also respond to external (outside our body) cues, whether that be particular times of the day (breakfast time, noon, and dinner time) or particular places (our kitchen, the movie theater), or particular activities (snacking while on a road trip). When that time or that place or that sight comes around, our hunger rises, just like Pavlov's dogs'.

Our external cues can be

- **environmental**—our physical and cultural surroundings, including standard mealtimes, ubiquitous coffee shops, and advertising;
- **cognitive**—the thoughts we associate with food;
- **emotional**—boredom or stress or sadness; and/or
- **social**—our friends, families, or colleagues talking about, eating, or offering food.

Conditioned hunger is a physiological response to repeated associations. External food cues can make us hungry, lead us to overeat, encourage us to eat UPFs, and derail our weight-loss goals. The more aware we can become of the food cues that lead us to eat, the more we can break the cycle of conditioned hunger.

ENVIRONMENTAL FOOD CUES

ENVIRONMENTAL FOOD CUES are subtle yet powerful triggers in our surroundings that influence our eating behavior, often without conscious awareness. Understanding these cues can be the key to making informed food choices.

Eating by the clock

Over an average day, the hunger hormone ghrelin spikes three times: slightly before breakfast, and again before lunch and dinner (Figure 10.1[2]). This rise is not a coincidence;[3] it is a conditioned response. If you normally eat three times a day, you will get hungry three times a day. If you normally eat six times a day, you'll get hungry six times a day.

Figure 10.1. The rise in ghrelin to signal hunger is a learned behavior that coincides with when we usually eat

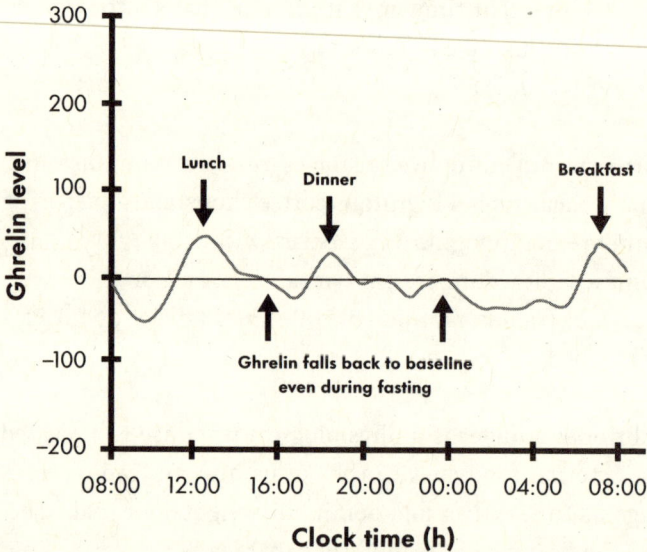

Conditioned hunger has become a big problem because Americans are eating more often than ever before. Instead of the three times a day that was usual in the 1970s, the average American is now eating more than five times per day (2.8 meals and 2.3 snacks per day).[4] This increased frequency of eating means they'll spike their ghrelin and feel hunger more frequently too.

The more we eat (or expect to eat), the more often we feel hungry. The idea of eating six appetizer-sized "meals" daily to make us hungry and then relying on our willpower to stop eating before we are full *sounds* stupid because it *is* stupid. "Grazing" is an effective eating strategy for cows, but not for humans.

Snacking is, by definition, an unnecessary food eaten between meals. This makes snack food an indulgence, not a necessity—and certainly not healthy or beneficial for weight loss. **There is no such thing as a healthy snack.** Healthy snacks are a contradiction, an oxymoron, like jumbo shrimp.

Remember that we are all individuals. For some people, eating multiple times daily can work. If it does, then keep doing what you are doing. However, if it does not, then don't feel obligated to continue grazing. That's the point. Eating constantly is not physiologically necessary. Our body stores food energy (calories) as body fat, which exists precisely so that we do **not** need to eat constantly. Who loves when you eat all the time? The food companies that make UPFs. Perhaps that explains why eating constantly is so heavily promoted.

For most of us, eating constantly is a nuisance. When are you supposed to get your work done if you are endlessly thinking about what you need to eat and when to eat it? If you want to lose weight, you want to think **less** about food, not more. And yet the irony is that if you are always eating, you'll want to continue eating. That's bad. If you are not eating, keep not eating. That's good. Inertia can either work for you or against you.

I've noticed many times that I wasn't hungry, but I ate anyway, usually for a social reason. As I began eating, my appetite returned, and I finished the entire meal relatively normally. Before eating, I could have happily skipped that meal. Once I started eating, I ate everything on my plate. The first few bites whet my appetite. Eating when you are not hungry is not a winning strategy for weight loss.

If you normally eat only once or twice a day, you only get hungry once or twice a day, since you aren't expecting to eat. Getting hungry less often? That's a huge, huge advantage for weight loss. The problem is controlling the hunger, not the calories. Managing hunger that comes twice a day is a lot easier than managing hunger that comes six times per day.

Tip #39: Don't eat all the time.
Give your body a chance to use the calories you have eaten.

At the same time that we're eating more often, fasting has been heavily discouraged. Eating less often and fasting more often are simply two sides of the same coin. It's the same thing. Skipping a meal? Hoo boy, those are fighting words. Eating frequently is supposed to stabilize our blood glucose levels, increase satiety, prevent hunger, and prevent overeating. But no scientific studies actually support this belief,[5] and logic argues against it.

What happens if you skip a meal? The graph that shows our ghrelin levels throughout the day reveals an important clue (see Figure 10.1). If you skip a meal, ghrelin does *not* continuously increase. It simply goes back down to baseline. After the initial wave, hunger recedes. Ghrelin shows a "spontaneous decrease after approximately 2 hours without food consumption."[6] Think about a time when you were busy and worked right through lunch. At about 1:00 p.m. you were hungry, but by 3:00 p.m., you were no longer hungry and probably felt normal. If you get hungry between meals, you don't need to snack. If you simply ignore it, the hunger will naturally fade away.

What happened? When you didn't eat, your body took the energy (calories) it needed from stored sources—blood sugar or body fat. When you don't eat a meal, you "eat" your body fat. Hunger goes down and body fat is reduced. Perfect! Your body carries fat (stored calories) precisely so that you have a source of calories if you don't eat. You should use body fat for what it is designed for.

Knowing that the hunger is temporary helps you deal with it. People are intimidated when they fast or skip a meal because they expect their hunger to keep building until they can't stand it anymore. But hunger recedes when you ignore it. Hunger comes in a wave and will eventually pass. Ride the waves; they will pass.

Ghrelin rises when your stomach is empty and falls when it is filled. That pattern is often the justification for constant eating. But there is another way to reduce ghrelin. Leave the stomach empty long enough, and ghrelin will eventually go down. In other words, stop eating long enough to build this practice into a habit, and the clock stops being a stimulus for the conditioned response of hunger.

Interestingly, when you fast for several days, ghrelin continues to drop. Ghrelin levels are about 25 percent lower than normal after three days of fasting.[7] As your body continues to "feed" itself with body fat, hunger diminishes. Ghrelin is lower. You are less hungry. The longer you fast, the easier it gets.

Many of my patients have experienced this phenomenon. They expect to be ravenously hungry after fasting but discover after a while that their hunger has receded. For example, one young doctor at our clinic had been overweight his whole life, and he felt like food controlled him. I encouraged him to try a fast of several days. He was nervous about feeling hungry but decided to give fasting a try. Afterward, he said: "For the first time in my life I turned down food because I just didn't want it. It wasn't that I was abstaining because I was fasting, I just really wasn't hungry. I've never turned down food like that before." He ate less but felt more full. Why? His body was eating stored calories (body fat). Perfect.

Finishing everything on the plate

We, as adults, flatter ourselves by imagining that we eat to get enough vital nutrients. That's generally false. Mostly we eat depending on the clock and other external cues, like how much food is put on our plate.

Children stop eating when they are full, no matter how much food we give them. They listen to their natural hunger and satiety signaling (homeostatic hunger). That's why it's sometimes so hard to get toddlers to eat at mealtimes. Parents often chase their children around the room with forkfuls of food. But as kids grow up, we teach them to ignore their body's natural satiety signals. Kids learn to eat at specific times, whether hungry or not. They learn to eat everything on their plate, hungry or not.

This belief that we should always finish what's on our plate is a bigger problem as portion sizes increase. The portion sizes of recipes in recent editions of classic cookbooks are much larger than the originals. Servings of french fries, hamburgers, and sodas are two to three times what they were in the 1970s.[8] The typical cheeseburger in the early 1990s was 4.5 oz (128 grams). Today's burger is 8 oz (227 grams). A bagel measured 3 inches (7.6 cm) in diameter in the 1990s. Today's bagel is 6 inches (15.2 cm) across.[9] A bottle of Coke in 1960 was 6.5 oz (192 ml). Today's Double Big Gulp from 7-Eleven is almost ten times larger, at 64 oz (1.9 L).

If you order a cheeseburger meal, you'll likely finish it all—whether today or in the 1990s. That's for two reasons: first, the expectation effect (you assume a portion is the appropriate size; see page 174) and second, the pressure to conform to societal norms (you feel you should finish your plate of food). Yet today, you'd be eating more than twice as much as in the 1990s to achieve the same level of satiety. We hardly notice when Supersized meals and Big Gulp drinks get bigger. Restaurants market them as "value meals" and carmakers just install larger cup holders, which normalizes these mega-sized portions.

Our perceptions and cultural norms, not our physiology, are most responsible for how much we eat. Restaurant portions in Europe and Japan are considerably smaller than those in the U.S.[10] And while people in both France and the U.S. will usually eat one portion of food and feel just as full, the portion in France is much smaller. The external cue (the empty plate) signifies the end of the meal, so the French do not feel hungry. But they've eaten much less to reduce that hunger, which translates into an overall reduced body weight.

Knowing that a full plate will encourage you to eat more, you can use different strategies to eat less. For example, you might use smaller plates and reduce the portion sizes of food. You might also skip the appetizer course. People typically eat all of their main course, whether they ate an appetizer or not, and feel equally satiated. Even the name "appetizer"—a small, tasty morsel to stimulate our hunger—gives away its role in weight gain. If you are trying to lose weight, why would you want to increase your appetite?

> **Tip #40:** Aim for fewer courses per meal, no snacks between or after meals, and smaller plates and portions.

Eating on the go

More and more, modern living seems to be about maximizing time. Typically, we rush from one meeting to another, or from home to the office to the gym, and we cram in food as we go. Often, this time crunch means poor food choices and rushed meals. The companies that make UPFs would have us believe that energy bars, microwaveable meals, and just-add-water mixes are the solution to our busy lives. In fact, eating quickly is a surefire recipe for hunger and for weight gain.

In the Chinese tradition, special occasions are often celebrated with a ten-course meal that can last for hours. The meal takes so long that I am usually full by the end of the third course. That feeling of satiety is simply a conditioned response because my meals typically last thirty minutes or so. Once past that time, my appetite shuts down because I expect the meal to be over. I'm full, and ready to get up and leave.

Use this conditioned response to your advantage in a busy day by eating slowly. Eating slowly decreases ghrelin and increases peptide YY, which translates into increased fullness that reduces future snacking by 25 percent.[11] Eating quickly leads to higher insulin (bad) and lower levels of the satiety hormones peptide YY and GLP-1 (also bad).

Eating slowly is even more important when eating energy-dense foods like UPFs.[12] When foods are bulky or more difficult to eat, like leafy greens and fibrous vegetables, we have no choice but to slow down to eat them. In contrast, UPFs are notoriously easy to eat, which makes them quick to eat as well. UPFs practically dissolve in your mouth (cheese puffs, commercial white bread, cereal bars). Consider the difference between eating sunflower seeds in their shell and sunflower seeds that have been shelled, roasted, salted, and sometimes flavored. Which would you eat more of?

People who eat slowly eat less and feel more full after.[13] Eat less, but feel more full? Sounds like a good strategy for weight loss to me.

Ultra-processed foods are designed to be extremely easy and quick to eat. They're often "pre-digested" in some way, either through processing or through the addition of chemicals such as emulsifiers and texturizers. They are essentially a form of adult baby food. When foods are easy and quick to eat, we eat more, so companies sell more and make more money.

Tip #41: Eat slowly. Take small bites and chew thoroughly. Don't wolf down your food.

COGNITIVE AND SENSORY FOOD CUES

AS WE'VE SEEN, the combination of cognitive (brain) and sensory (body) cues can be very potent in obesogenic environments. Food manufacturers and food marketers use a variety of sights and smells to make us think about food all the time. As individuals, we internalize these cues as a constant expectation for food. This expectation effect is a conditioned response.

Our expectations around food

Expectation is a huge part of conditioned hunger. In some cases, our expectations make us more hungry; in other cases, less hungry.

In medicine, we know that the placebo effect is both real and powerful. Sham surgery, for example, when a surgeon only makes an incision and sutures it back up, performs about 70 percent as well as real bariatric surgery. The weight loss experienced by patients with sham surgery is derived merely from the expectation of the "surgery."[14] The weight loss is real, but the mechanism for losing the weight lies mostly within the mind, not the stomach.

Similarly, often the expectation of eating, and not necessarily the food energy (calories) itself, can trigger hunger or satiety. In one study, researchers gave two groups an identical 380-calorie milkshake. They told one group it was an "indulgent" 620-calorie milkshake, and the other, a "sensible" 140-calorie milkshake. Ghrelin levels dropped more when people thought they were drinking the higher-calorie shake.[15] The expectation effect is the reason that sham feeding, where food is chewed but then spit out, also decreases hunger and ghrelin, even though no calories are ingested.[16]

Eating "diet" foods, "lean" cuisine, or meal replacement shakes is a fool's game because of this conditioned expectation effect. That doesn't stop food companies from marketing foods this way, however. You don't expect those foods to make you full, so they won't. Eventually your hunger will win out, and you'll just stop "dieting." Yes, those "diet" foods have fewer calories. But why don't they help with weight loss? Because it's the hunger that's the problem, not the calories. When foods are labeled "healthy" or "lite," we adopt a deprivation mindset and expect that they won't taste good or fill us up. This expectation becomes a self-fulfilling prophecy.

Several studies show this effect to be real. People who ate a protein bar labeled "healthy" were 60 percent hungrier than those eating the same bar labeled "yummy." In fact, people who thought they were eating a "healthy" snack were hungrier than if they ate nothing at all![17] Similarly, people eat 30 percent more vegetables when the vegetables are given tasty-sounding names like Bang Bang Broccoli and Zesty Sweet Potato.[18] In another example, participants in a study felt less full after eating a breakfast labeled as "250-calorie sensible" compared with "500-calorie indulgent." Both breakfasts were identical except for the label.[19]

Expected satiety influences how much you eat overall. In one experiment, participants ate a three-egg omelet but were shown an ingredient list with either two eggs and 30 grams (1.1 oz) of cheese or four eggs and 60 grams (2.2 oz) of cheese. Participants who believed they ate the larger meal had lower hunger ratings through the day and also ate less overall that day (167 calories less).[20]

To lose weight, we need to change eating behavior. This means we need to pay attention to the cues that compel us to eat, our conditioned responses, and the expectation effect. Again, to reduce hunger, reduce the mention and expectation of food.

> **Tip #42:** Avoid the expectation effect and deprivation mindset. Don't eat food specifically labeled "diet" or "sensible" or "healthy."

EMOTIONAL FOOD CUES

EMOTIONAL FOOD CUES, such as boredom, anxiety, sadness, and joy, are internal triggers that prompt people to eat. The food is meant to satisfy or regulate emotions rather than physical hunger or the need for nutrients. Unlike environmental food cues, emotional food cues are deeply tied to personal experiences, cultural associations, and learned behaviors. We've covered many of these in the section on hedonic hunger, so I will only briefly discuss boredom.

Eating out of boredom

When nothing else is going on, what is more enjoyable than getting together with friends for a bite to eat? After all, eating is a perfectly socially acceptable reason that everybody can relate to. But are you really hungry, or simply bored? Likewise, when you are scheduled to go out to dinner or to a bar with friends or family, you may find yourself eating when you aren't particularly hungry.

Find other ways to socialize. Schedule walks, plan social sports like tennis or golf, join a knitting circle. Go outside and sit on a bench. Hiking in the woods or along a nature trail increases activity in your sympathetic nervous system, which suppresses hunger. Inviting friends to join you increases the pleasure of the walk and can take your mind off food. Being in nature helps calm and relax you—and leave the triggering food environment behind.

176

> **Tip #43:** To take your mind off food, be busy.
> Choose a hobby. Go outside. Call your friends.

SOCIAL FOOD CUES

SOCIAL FOOD CUES come from other people, either directly or indirectly. Some of these cues are societal, as we saw in Chapter 9. For example, the social and cultural norms in our country, region, or city influence our individual decisions. Many of these social cues, though, come from our immediate friends and family. Here are a couple of common social cues that we internalize as habits, or conditioned hunger.

Celebrating (and relaxing) with food

Almost every culture celebrates with food, and most people celebrate many times a year. Families and friends gather to celebrate birthdays, christenings, graduations, weddings, family reunions, funerals, and more. Work colleagues celebrate promotions, profit sharing, retirements, meeting goals. Faith communities celebrate holy days. Virtually all of these major events involve at least one special meal, and often food and alcohol flow almost constantly. In any given year, people gain most of their weight during celebrations and vacations.

Americans experience most of their yearly weight gain between Thanksgiving and the New Year. The Japanese tend to gain weight over Golden Week, and the Germans gain weight at Christmas and Easter.[21] While some of this weight gain is lost over the ensuing months, about half persists. Vacations—think ocean cruises, all-inclusive resorts, and summer cottages where the day seems to be one continuous stream of fattening snacks, meals, and alcoholic drinks—are also associated with a weight gain of 0.32 kg (0.7 pounds), most of which is not lost even six weeks afterward.[22]

If you plan to eat heavily during a celebration or vacation, I advise people to eat very strictly for a week before or after, with increased fasting and no indulgences. For example, I eat guilt-free during the

177

week of a celebration or vacation but know that I'll be paying the tab at the end. I fast more the week after a festive period or vacation, until my pants start fitting normally again. If the timing doesn't work out to fast after my vacation, I'll fast more the week before. Balance: this idea is not new or original. In the Christian tradition of Lent, people eat less or fast leading up to Easter, which is marked by celebration and feasting.

Alternatively, cultivate some new social traditions that don't involve food or that involve healthier foods. Play games or go for a walk together instead of baking cookies. Plan a couple of side dishes instead of a dozen, and include some leafy greens instead of carbs. Keep green tea, coffee, and sparkling water on hand instead of beer, wine, and spirits.

> **Tip #44:** Manage weight gain during celebrations and vacations by planning a week of strict eating or fasting to balance each week of holiday.

Eating out

In the 1970s, virtually no one ate at a restaurant every week. By the 1990s and 2000s, some people were meeting with clients or colleagues in a restaurant, cafeteria, or bar every day of the week. While a three-martini lunch may be good for business relations, it's definitely not good for your weight. Even without the alcohol, grabbing lunch at the local diner every day—especially if the specials are a constant rotation of comfort foods—will significantly increase your weight. If you immediately associate business meetings with the bar, or lunch with colleagues at the diner, you may want to rethink these habits. Restaurants prioritize taste and price, not your waistline.

Plan ahead. Consider a walking meeting, or meet in a place that doesn't serve food or alcohol. Pack a homemade lunch and encourage your colleagues to do the same, then eat in a local park. If you eat out, choose a place with healthier food options. If portions are large, split one portion with a friend. Or bring a take-home container and put half of the food in the container before you start to eat. Instead of ordering food in for work events, ask everyone to bring a salad or vegetable dish to share with one or two other people.

> **Tip #45:** Eat homemade as much as possible, since you often don't know how restaurant or takeout foods are prepared.

HOW TO COUNTER CONDITIONED HUNGER

THE UNDERLYING PREMISE of most diets and "expert" guidance is that your weight is your own fault, since you decide what you eat. But this misses the overriding importance of environmental—societal and social—factors. Yes, you can decide if you will eat or not, but you cannot decide if you will be *hungry* or not. And today's obesogenic environment and social norms condition you to be hungry all the time.

Here's the big problem. You, my friend, are Pavlov's dog. Think about it this way. A bell rings. *Ding!* Dogs generally don't care. But Pavlov's dogs react to the cue, and their conditioned response is to get hungry and start salivating immediately. That's not their fault. That's their conditioning. Now think about the human equivalent.

You wake up. *Ding!* "Breakfast time." You get hungry.

The time is noon. *Ding!* "Lunchtime." You get hungry.

You finish work. *Ding!* "Dinnertime." You get hungry.

Your plate is full. *Ding!* "You must finish everything on your plate," even though it's clearly too much food.

You get some coffee. *Ding!* "You need a muffin." You get hungry.

You're in a work meeting. *Ding!* "You need a cookie." You get hungry.

The time is 4:00 p.m. *Ding!* "You need a snack." You get hungry.

You get in your car. *Ding!* "You need some drive-thru." You get hungry.

You go to the mall. *Ding!* "You see and smell the food court." You get hungry.

179

You go to the movies with friends. *Ding!* "You need popcorn." You get hungry.

You watch TV before bed, when food shows and food advertising are frequent. *Ding!* "You think about food." You get hungry.

Then some "genius" comes along and says: "Oh, you are gaining weight because you are eating too much. Just eat less. Calories In, Calories Out, you know." But notice that they never tell you how to **deal with the hunger**.

Once the neutral stimulus (for example, a bell) is conditioned to the expectation of food, how do you get rid of it? Behavioral science reveals two strategies: extinction and counterconditioning.

Extinction means ringing a bell repeatedly but not giving food. Eventually the expectation of food disappears. Counterconditioning means pairing the bell to a new, different noxious response, such as an electric shock. Again, the expectation of food eventually disappears.

Luckily for us, extinction and counterconditioning are almost equally effective,[23] so I won't be recommending the electric cattle prod in *The Obesity Code* book series. Yet.

To extinguish the conditioned hunger response to these many cues to eating in daily life, we need to turn to an ancient practice: fasting. The secret to automatic and lasting weight loss is changing our default setting from eating to not eating. That's where a structured eating day, fasting, and positive mindset and healthy habits come in. Whether the root cause of your hunger is homeostatic, hedonic, conditioned, or a combination, the strategies in Part 4 will help you lose weight. More importantly, they will also help you to keep it off.

JAMAL

Jamal had been severely overweight his entire life, and he started every diet believing he would fail. And with that mindset, he did. Every time he regained the weight he'd lost, his belief that he was "doomed" to obesity was reinforced. He bought clothes simply because they fit, avoided cameras, felt ashamed in public, and dreaded stairs.

When Jamal joined The Fasting Method, we worked to help him change not only the foods he was eating and when but also his attitude toward food. For Jamal, it was his thoughts, feelings, beliefs, and environment that were holding him back. For many months, he worked closely with lifestyle coaches, learned about eating whole foods and intermittent fasting, and found an accountability partner to support his journey. He moved slowly and intentionally: he didn't just want to be thin, he wanted to become a healthy person with a healthy identity.

Today, at fifty-seven, he's lost 85 pounds (39 kg), reversed fatty liver and prediabetes, and has a positive relationship with food. Jamal says he's become a different person—not just on the outside, but on the inside too.

SARIKA

When Sarika decided to have children, her doctor suggested she lose some weight and get healthy before getting pregnant. Sarika had recently injured her ankle and so she focused her weight-loss efforts on fasting rather than exercise. She began to fast consistently, sometimes alternating days, sometimes eating one or two meals a day, and occasionally fasting for up to seventy-two hours. Over nine months, Sarika lost 70 pounds (32 kg).

To keep the weight off, she's learned to stay consistent, through all of life's challenges. The most important keys to her success have been getting community support to help her stay on track, shifting her mindset, and changing her habits.

Sarika is feeling strong and healthy, and she's expecting her first child! She looks forward to returning to fasting after her child is born.

BARB

Barb had been heavy her whole life, and she had been trying to lose weight for just as long. By age forty, she had tried every diet. She'd have some success but then always gained back all the weight. She had even tried intermittent fasting and lost 25 pounds (11 kg), but again she gained back all the weight. As a health care professional, she thought she understood how to lose weight. Knowledge alone, however, is not enough to create behavior change. Often it takes a community.

Barb knew that high insulin was the root cause of her weight gain. She knew that a low-carbohydrate diet helped her lose weight and feel better. But she couldn't shake her hunger. Working with a lifestyle coach, committing to fasting consistently, and seeking support from others on their own weight-loss journeys finally made the difference.

Barb began to look on her fasting as she would a treatment for a life-threatening illness. She started following a low-carb eating plan and doing alternate-day fasting with no exceptions. Six months later, she had lost 55 pounds (25 kg)—more weight than she had ever managed to lose before. Her sleep apnea and pre-diabetes resolved.

Three years later, Barb has lost 80 pounds (36 kg) and kept it off, and she now supports others on their own weight-loss journeys.

PART
FOUR

How to Manage Hunger

MAKING
WEIGHT LOSS AUTOMATIC

MAGINE THAT IT'S the 1970s and you are stuck in a mid-afternoon meeting. You're bored and would like a snack to pass the time. There's no coffee shop in the building, the cafeteria is closed after lunch, and there's nowhere within walking distance that sells coffee. You have to leave the meeting, get your car, and drive around to find a shop to sell you a coffee and a cookie. If you can get the coffee to go, which is not a given, you have to hold it to avoid spilling as you drive because there's no cup holder in the car. When you get back to the meeting, your boss stares at you, wondering where the hell you've been for the last forty-five minutes and whether to fire your sorry ass. Would you actually do this? Unlikely.

In this 1970s scenario, it isn't willpower that prevents you from taking off for coffee and a cookie in the middle of the meeting. It's the default condition of not eating. It takes a lot of willpower to snack, and no will-power to *not* snack. The social environment shapes your eating behavior.

Now let's replay this situation in the 2020s. You're in a mid-afternoon meeting and a colleague has ordered a plate of cookies and a pot of coffee for the group. You're not really hungry but you *are* really bored. So, you eat two cookies to pass the time. You hardly notice you're doing it. In fact, it takes massive willpower to *not* eat the cookies that you don't particularly want or need.

What's the difference? It's not the lack of knowledge. It's not our emotions. Our eating day has no structure, and without structure, we default to "eat all the time."

The "experts" tell you that you can eat whatever, whenever, wherever, and however much you want, if the total calories are controlled. Our society and our social norms have changed to accommodate this new default of "eat all the time." The modern "scientific" advice gives no structure—the what, when, where, why, and how much to eat—to scaffold a proper diet.

Structure is important for many realms, not just weight loss. For example, imagine that you'd like to run a marathon, so you hire a coach. Your coach sets out a detailed training plan for every week: how far, how fast, how long you'll run; the foods you'll eat; the different workouts (interval training, sprints) you'll do. Your friend hires a different "expert" whose training plan leaves it up to your friend to do whatever training they want, as long as they run the full marathon at the end. Who do you imagine will do better?

STRUCTURE THE EATING DAY

THE STRUCTURE OF the eating day is the framework for your dietary plan. In the 1970s, what, when, where, why, and how much you ate followed a very rigid, defined structure.

- **What** did you eat? Whatever your mom or dad cooked, usually natural whole foods cooked traditionally. Eating out was rare, and McDonald's was a once-a-year treat at best. Boxed or pre-packaged foods didn't dominate the kitchen.
- **When** did you eat? You ate three meals per day: breakfast, lunch, and dinner, with no snacks allowed. If you wanted something to

eat after school, your mom said: "No, you'll ruin your dinner." If you wanted a bedtime snack, your mom said: "No, you should have eaten more at dinner."

- **Where** did you eat? You could eat in the kitchen, the dining room, or the cafeteria. That's it. No eating in front of the TV. No eating in your room. No eating at your desk. No eating while playing games. No eating during sports. No eating in front of the computer.
- **Why** did you eat? Mainly to satisfy hunger. Without many ultra-processed foods, emotional eating and food addiction were rare. Since you couldn't eat wherever you wanted, eating out of boredom was more difficult. Food networks showing food twenty-four hours a day did not exist. Cooking shows taught people how to cook. They weren't a competition, a reality show, or entertainment.
- **How much** did you eat? Whatever was on your plate. But 1970s portion sizes were one-half to one-third as large as today's portions, because food was much more expensive.

The default 1970s-era eating schedule allows a very narrow range of possibilities. When the default is "not eating," you have to make a real effort to break this social and societal norm that is constantly reinforced. Obesity, as you might expect, was relatively rare. Today, that default may be hard to imagine, but was this eating schedule difficult for people to follow at the time? Did not eating take a lot of willpower? Not at all, because it was just the way things were. The default was the same for everybody you knew. It was just life as everybody knew it.

For some odd reason, the scientific consensus is that a structured eating plan is not necessary for weight loss, unlike virtually every other human endeavor. All that is necessary is to count calories. When this approach fails, the experts blame the victim. We will review these questions in more detail in Chapter 13.

189

> **Tip #46:** To lose weight automatically, give your eating day some structure: breakfast, lunch, and dinner, no snacks.

If you have the authority, you might institute some simple changes at the workplace.

- No food at meetings.
- Eating is allowed in the cafeteria only. A desk is for working, not eating.
- No cakes or other food for celebrations in the office.
- No bowls of candy on desks.
- No cookies or donuts or other snack items in the office area.
- Bring back the water cooler.

Eating cakes, cookies, and candies in the office is unfair to anyone trying to lose weight or maintain their health. That is reason enough to make changes.

MAKE NOT EATING YOUR DEFAULT SETTING

I SUBSCRIBE TO three daily newspapers and four newsletters. You know why? I rationalize that I'm simply well read, but I'm really just a sucker. The reason I have all these subscriptions is because after the trial periods ran out, I was not motivated enough to cancel. When we don't know or don't want to think about what to do, we simply take the choice that's already been made for us. And as most businesses know, the best way to keep customers on is to make the default setting an automatic renewal. Inertia is powerful.

What does the default setting mean for weight loss? **Everything.**

In the 1970s, weight loss was almost automatic. People didn't diet much and hardly exercised, yet obesity was still rare. Why? The default setting was "**not eating.**" People ate a few meals at specific times in specific places and for a specific purpose. And people ate specific foods: usually natural foods cooked at home. Snacks and eating between meals were rare, and most days included a lengthy fasting period. If you were eating, you were eating. If you were doing something else (watching TV, driving, working at your desk), then you weren't eating.

The key to automatic weight loss is not willpower. It's not knowledge. It's not skill. The key is your default setting. Is your default to eat natural, unprocessed foods or junk food? Is your default to eat three times a day or six? Is your default to fast for twelve to fourteen hours every day, or only while you're asleep? Is your default to drink water or sugary sodas?

The seemingly trivial decisions about your default settings make a massive difference in your success or failure to lose weight.

FAST EVERY DAY

THE DIET OF 1970s America included a lot of white bread and jam, ice cream, and Oreo cookies. I grew up in the 1970s. We were *not* eating whole-wheat bread or pasta. We were *not* eating quinoa. We were *not* eating kale. We were *not* counting calories. We were *not* counting carbs. We were *not* even really exercising much. We were doing everything "wrong" and yet, seemingly effortlessly, there was no obesity. Why?

The answer, again, is: **We were not eating all the time.**

The National Health and Nutrition Examination Survey found that in 1977, most Americans ate three times per day: breakfast, lunch, and dinner. Snacks were not considered either necessary or healthy. They were treats, to be had only very occasionally. The result was that Americans were fasting daily, from after dinner until breakfast the next morning. This break of twelve to fourteen hours or more allowed blood glucose and insulin to fall and the body to release stored energy (burn fat) every single day.

By 2004, however, most people were eating almost six times per day: breakfast, lunch, and dinner, plus snacks in between. The fasting period started to shrink, meaning that blood glucose and insulin remained higher throughout the day and the body had less time to burn off extra fat energy between the after-dinner snack and breakfast the next morning.

Today, it is considered unconscionable to skip the mid-morning or after-school snack. When my kids were younger and played soccer, parents brought snacks to eat between the halves of the game. We begged the kids to eat their cookies and drink their juice. Then we wondered why we have a childhood obesity crisis. Good job, everybody, good job.

More recently, as incomes have increased and more Western products have become available, China has followed in America's footsteps with increased snacking. In 1991, only 8.7 percent of Chinese children snacked regularly. By 2009, that number was up to 46.3 percent, a rise of more than 500 percent. The rise in snacking among adults was similar, from 8.7 percent to 35.6 percent.[1] Obesity rates have skyrocketed in China along with the snacking.

Today, the span of time in which Americans eat each day is fourteen and three-quarter hours. If you ate breakfast at 9 a.m., on average you didn't stop eating until 11:45 p.m.! Practically the only time people don't eat is while sleeping.[2] And we are sleeping fewer hours every night. People are also eating later and later, with an estimated 35 percent of calories consumed after 6 p.m. This eating pattern is problematic if you are trying to lose weight. A small fasting window due to eating late (increased insulin) and getting too little sleep (increased ghrelin) is a recipe for weight gain. When people were instructed to use early time-restricted eating, meaning that they ate within an eight-hour window between 7 a.m. and 3 p.m., they lost far more weight compared to eating over the standard twelve hours or more.[3]

Why did we start to snack more and eat more often? Because we were hungry! The foods we were eating no longer kept us full. It was not a deliberate choice.

In the 1970s, we might have eaten two eggs and ham for breakfast, which kept us full until lunchtime. By the 1980s, low-fat boxed cereal, white bread and jam, and a glass of orange juice had become the new breakfast of choice (and "champions"). But those ultra-processed foods, devoid of protein or fat for satiety, couldn't keep us full until lunch. By mid-morning, we were desperately looking around for a low-fat muffin to stave off the hunger pangs and tide us through to lunch.

In the 1970s, we might have eaten a bowl of soup and leftover meat-loaf for lunch. By the 1980s, that lunch was more likely a white bread sandwich with processed meat, plus cookies and a soda pop. Once again, this ultra-processed lunch with little protein or fat for satiety couldn't keep us full. By mid-afternoon, we were hungry and looking for cookies or a chocolate bar or a bag of chips to patch us through to dinner. After dinner, it was the same story all over again.

Now, instead of eating three times per day, we were eating six times per day. What we eat determines how often and how much we eat, through the mechanism of satiety. Because the U.S.'s new dietary guidelines extolled low-fat, low-calorie foods, we began to eat an ultra-processed food diet high in refined carbohydrates that made us so hungry that we thought that eating six times a day was good for us. But it wasn't. And yet many of us still eat this way today.

The time you spend fasting is critical, because that is the only time your body burns fat. When you are eating, you can't burn fat. Fat burning only happens when you don't eat (fasting).

The difference between the fed state and the fasted state

In *The Obesity Code*, we discussed the critical difference between when our body is storing energy (the fed state) and when it is burning energy (the fasted state). That difference is worth reviewing here, because it helps us to understand exactly why daily fasting is such an important part of weight loss. If we don't stop eating all the time, we can't lose weight.

Body fat is simply a store of calories. When we eat, insulin goes up, which tells our body to store calories (as body fat). When we don't eat (fasting), insulin goes down, which tells our body to burn those stored calories (body fat). The human body exists in one of two states: the fed state (insulin high, storing calories) and the fasted state (insulin low, burning calories). The body is either **storing** food energy or **burning** stored food energy but not both at the same time (Table 11.1).

193

Table 11.1. The body exists in two states: fed or fasted

The fed state (insulin high)	The fasted state (insulin low)
Store calories (as body fat)	Burn stored calories (body fat)
Don't burn calories	Don't store calories

When we eat, insulin goes up, which stimulates de novo lipogenesis (the creation of new fat stores) and glycogen synthesis (the creation of new glycogen, or sugar stores). This is a fancy way to say that when insulin is high, we store the incoming calories as fat or sugar. High insulin also inhibits lipolysis and glycogenolysis, which is a fancy way of saying that when insulin is high, the body cannot burn stored fat or sugar (glycogen). This mechanism makes sense. When we are eating, we want to store some of the calories for later on.

What happens if insulin levels are excessively high? That's not hard to predict. Don't overthink things.

- Insulin tells our body to store sugar. If insulin is too high, we store too much sugar. This is the disease known as type 2 diabetes.
- Insulin tells our body to store fat. If insulin is too high, we store too much fat. This is the disease known as obesity.

Insulin is not "bad." It is a natural hormone doing its given job. But excessive levels of any hormone can cause disease. Our ability to store food energy (calories) is the reason we don't die in our sleep every single night. When we're not eating, such as during sleep, our body still requires energy for basic metabolism (brain, heart, kidneys, and so on), and that food energy (calories) must come from storage (sugar or fat). **The trigger is not excess calories. The trigger is insulin.** If you eat six times a day, you spike insulin six times a day, which tells your body "Please put calories into body fat" six times a day. That is a recipe for heartbreak and heartburn.

Fasting is simply the fastest and most efficient method of reducing insulin (Figure 11.1), which is very beneficial if insulin levels are high, as they are in people with excess weight, pre-diabetes, or type 2 diabetes. Calorie restriction does not necessarily lower insulin levels. This is why fasting succeeds where calorie restriction sometimes fails. Adjusting our eating behavior to lower insulin, as detailed in Part 1, also helps.

Figure 11.1. Eating increases insulin and food energy storage (body fat) whereas fasting decreases insulin and body fat

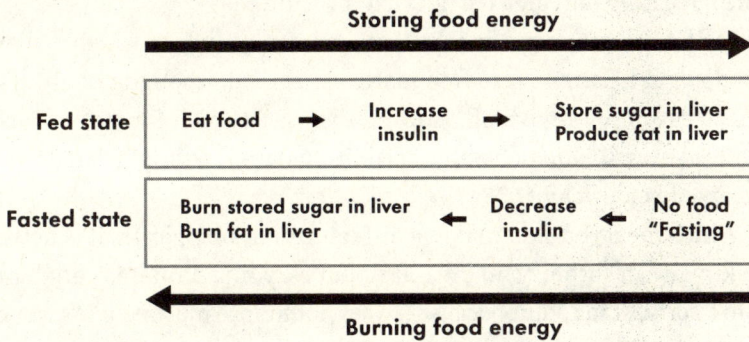

Storing food energy →

Fed state	Eat food ➡	Increase insulin ➡	Store sugar in liver Produce fat in liver

Fasted state	Burn stored sugar in liver Burn fat in liver	⬅ Decrease insulin	⬅ No food "Fasting"

← **Burning food energy**

Tip #47: Burn fat by switching between the *fed* state (eating food, high insulin) and the *fasted* state (not eating, low insulin). Fasting is the most efficient way to lower insulin.

The value of skipping a meal

It's good to skip a meal. If you don't eat, your body will simply take the calories it needs from its stored calories, body fat. In the 1970s, naughty children were often sent to bed without dinner. I didn't experience this punishment personally because I was a very good child, but the twenty-hour fast didn't cause any lasting physical or emotional harm. Yes, the kids were hungry, and hopefully learned their lesson, but skipping a meal wasn't unhealthy—even if it happened regularly.

Today, if you skip a meal, some people react like you just spit on the Pope. "Oh. My. God," I can hear them saying. "You must *always* eat

195

breakfast, even if it is a Krispy Kreme donut!" Or, "Oh. My. God. I can't believe you have been awake for almost two minutes and haven't started cramming food into your mouth. Call 9-1-1!" Oh, by the way— why can't you lose any weight?

Don't overcomplicate things. You can't burn body fat if you are eating. You can only burn body fat when you are *not* eating. There's no way around this super-obvious fact. To lose weight, you need to spend more time *not* eating (fasting). It's not that difficult.

Eating cannot cause weight loss. You can only lose weight when you don't eat. Eating more frequently generally (although not always) means eating more overall. In the Adventist Health Study-2, which involved over 50,000 people, each additional meal was associated with increased body weight.[4]

Which meal you skip makes a difference. Physiologically, it is better to skip dinner rather than breakfast. But skipping dinner is very hard from a social standpoint because it does not fit into most people's work/life schedule. So, socially, breakfast is the best meal to skip. It's a trade-off.

Remember inertia? We are naturally inclined to do what's easy and then keep doing it. If skipping a particular meal gets too hard socially, then we'll eventually stop. Trying to shoehorn an eating schedule into an incompatible life schedule is a surefire weight-loss disaster.

For this reason, I eat dinner with my family most nights and skip breakfast instead. We rarely eat breakfast together because we're often rushing to school or work. Skipping breakfast allows me to use a default eating schedule of two meals per day, instead of three. When I do eat breakfast, I feel really full, so I can't eat lunch. This is the power of a default setting with a lower number of meals per day. Eating twice a day is normal for me, and therefore does not require willpower or thought. Yes, it may be best to only eat breakfast and lunch, but that doesn't work for many people (including me), so eating lunch and dinner is a good option.

There's nothing wrong with eating breakfast. There's nothing wrong with *not* eating breakfast. Breakfast is technically the meal that breaks your fast, and you can break your fast anytime you like, not necessarily in the early morning. After all, does anybody get upset when you eat brunch instead of breakfast? No. The bottom line is you want to get a nice, long fasting period overnight to maximize the time you are allowing your body to use stored calories (body fat). To do that, ideally you'll avoid eating dinner too late whether or not you plan to skip breakfast.

The key mistake to avoid when skipping any meal is to avoid eating more at the next meal. If you skip breakfast, you are allowing your body to "eat" its stores of calories (body fat). If you then eat more at lunch, you'll undo much of the good you've done. Eat as normally as possible after skipping a meal.

> **Tip #48:** Fast regularly to set up your body's expectation to burn fat, which helps make weight loss automatic.

THE SECOND GOLDEN RULE: DON'T EAT ALL THE TIME. FAST REGULARLY.

Not all weight-loss tips are equal. Some rules are more important than others. Avoiding ultra-processed foods is so important in today's food environment that I've called it a Golden Rule (page 116). Similarly, fasting is very important for weight loss because you can only lose weight when you don't eat.

The benefits of fasting go far beyond reducing calories. Fasting helps to lower the body fat thermostat because it reduces insulin. As insulin drops, other hormones go up. Growth hormone rises, which helps preserve lean tissue. Sympathetic tone (including the hormone noradrenaline) rises, which reduces hunger. Long-term fasting also reduces ghrelin, the hunger hormone. Fasting gives the body a

197

break from the ultra-processed foods that create problems with food addictions and emotional eating. Abstinence, which is the hallmark of fasting, helps to interrupt physical and psychological cravings. Regular fasting changes our conditioned response to food from always eating to the automatic response of weight loss. Making fasting a habit can further our chances of weight-loss success. Fasting helps to manage physiological, emotional, and social hunger.

To lose weight and keep it off, stick to a regular eating schedule and eat less, less often. Be sure to build in a period of fasting Every. Single. Day. Aim for a minimum fasting period of twelve to fourteen hours, as was typical in the 1970s. If you are trying to lose weight, then feel free to increase this fasting period, with supervision by your health care practitioner, to twenty-four hours, thirty-six hours, forty-two hours, three days, five days, or up to seven days.

| 12 |

UNLOCKING THE SECRETS OF SUCCESS—YOUR MINDSET AND YOUR HABITS

YEARS AGO, I drank my coffee in the manner Canadians call a "double-double," which means coffee with two splashes of cream and two spoonfuls of sugar. As I understood more about nutrition (because medical school didn't teach me much), I started to think to myself, "Sugar is poison." With that change in mindset, I just didn't want so much sugar. I still drink plenty of coffee, but it's been more than twenty years since I put sugar in it.

Changing my thoughts (mindset) changed my feelings about sugar (revulsion), which changed my judgment (it's undesirable), which influenced my action (avoiding sugar). But that process *begins* with the mindset. If I had simply cut out sugar, I would have faced a mindset of deprivation. I would have thought, "The sweets are something I want but cannot have." With my "sugar is poison" mindset still active today, I don't *want* so much sugar, so it's *easy* to change my actions. I don't eat zero sugar, but I probably eat 75 percent less than I did as a child. Over time, these benefits build up. The key is that reducing sugar was not the product of willpower, but a product of a changed mindset.

Many of us obsess about what to eat, but we should be talking about how to think. Weight loss is not just about replacing bread with ground beef, cutting a few hundred calories per day, or cutting out sugar. If you think weight loss is all about the food and the calories, you will almost certainly fail. That approach has been done. No, it didn't work.

Successful weight loss doesn't just change your diet, it reprograms your ideas about food, cravings, hunger, self-image, addiction, habits, social modeling, peer group, mindfulness, emotional eating, and more. That's why the social and societal values that surround us are so critical. Successful weight loss starts with the proper mindset about why you are eating what you are eating. The problem is the hunger—homeostatic, hedonic, and conditioned—not the calories.

MANAGING YOUR MINDSET

MINDSET, HOW WE emotionally process experiences, is an important but underappreciated aspect of weight loss. Your mindset involves your thoughts and "self-talk" and acts like a lens through which you can see things in a positive, neutral, or negative light. Two people can experience the exact same event in opposite ways.

Why does it matter so much?

- Thoughts have the power to shape your feelings.
- Feelings have the power to shape your judgments.
- Judgments have the power to shape your actions (Figure 12.1).

Figure 12.1. Our thoughts affect our judgments and our actions

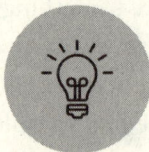

Thoughts
can shape
feelings

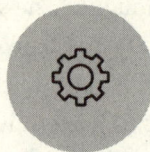

Feelings
can shape
judgments

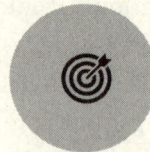

Judgments
can shape
actions

For example, suppose you have recently regained a bit of weight. Your mindset could tell you that you've failed, the weight gain is all your fault, and all the hard work you've done is wasted. You'll feel worthless, which will cause you to judge yourself harshly as a failure and a loser. This judgment will make you give up, eat some junk food, and swear to never try losing weight again.

Alternatively, your mindset could tell you that regaining a bit of weight is a normal part of the weight-loss journey, and maybe you need to refocus. Your thoughts give you a feeling of determination and hope that you'll do better. Your hopefulness causes you to judge yourself as being on track. Your judgment causes you to understand the root cause of your weight gain and work twice as hard to get your unruly weight back under control.

A negative mindset impairs your capacity for change and can easily trigger a persistent downward spiral. This negative mindset leads you to negative conclusions, and your actions reflect them.

Changing your mindset involves reframing your thoughts. While reframing takes a bit of work, it can literally change your life. Reframing involves deliberately pairing an event or item with your chosen mindset. This process will feel extremely artificial at first, but through repetition, it will feel more and more natural, until you actually believe your new mindset. Let's see how this process of reframing your thoughts might work.

Consider exercise. If your mindset is that exercise is a way to "work off" calories, then you'll never enjoy working out because it's pure drudgery. Your mindset is that exercise is a penance for eating good food. Exercise is not fun or healthy; it's just a grind. You will resent the time you spend exercising.

Instead, you could try to reframe exercise by thinking, "I am exercising because it is fun." At first, this statement won't seem right. However, each time you set out to exercise, you'll remind yourself that it's fun. And gradually, with that thought in your mind, you'll start to think that movement is a celebration of being alive. As you enjoy exercise more, you'll do more of it. Your mindset has allowed this change in your actions, which improves your health. Mindset is the key.

The popularity of smoking tobacco has gradually waned in America over the last few decades. In the 1960s, even though it was known to cause cancer and heart disease, smoking retained its popularity. Why? Because knowledge alone is not enough to affect behavior change. Only when the perception of smoking as "cool" changed to "dirty and disgusting" was real progress made. It all starts with mindset. The banning of tobacco advertising likely played a key role.

Here's the thing. If you think weight loss is all about *dietary* change, then you've already lost. The key to long-term successful weight loss is *behavior* change. That encompasses the knowledge of what and when to eat (homeostatic hunger), but also the emotional aspects (hedonic hunger) and the learned social and societal aspects of eating behavior (conditioned hunger).

How to develop a healthy mindset

A healthy mindset helps you to feel good about yourself. Instead of being a person who doesn't do things like exercise, eat healthy food, or set and reach goals, you become a person who does. You may not do all these things perfectly right away, but with a positive mindset you can achieve much more than you can with a negative mindset. Do your best to keep reframing negative thoughts. If you find yourself slipping back into a negative mindset, acknowledge that fact and recommit to your positive mindset.

Reframing your mindset is a two-step process:

1. Identify the mindset you'd like to reframe
2. Create a personal "mantra" for change

Let's consider two of the most important aspects of weight loss: avoiding ultra-processed foods and fasting regularly.

Reframing ultra-processed foods

Food companies have spent literally billions of dollars to associate their ultra-processed product with happy feelings. Coca-Cola associates their brand with Christmas, happiness, and family. Sugary cereals, Happy Meals, and candies portray fun with bright colors, licensed cartoon characters, and funny TV commercials. Since most of us have been watching these TV commercials since we were kids, these associations are ingrained. UPFs prompt us to think:

- It's fun.
- It's delicious.
- It's affordable.

To change your mindset, you must deliberately replace these automatic thoughts with a different message. Create a mantra, something you say to yourself to help change your mindset. For example, when you see a box of UPF, deliberately say or think to yourself:

- This is not real food. This is fake food, full of chemicals.
- This is ultra-addictive food that I should avoid.
- This is ultra-processed and therefore ultra-fattening. No thank you.

At first, this process seems unnatural. But slowly the mindset you've deliberately chosen will come to dominate and seem completely normal. This new mindset can completely change the way you feel about foods.

Deliberately changing my mindset helped me eat less sugar, and I use the same process for ultra-processed foods. When I walk into the grocery store and see boxes of prepared foods, I sometimes deliberately think to myself, "Gross, so ultra-processed," even if I happen to like a particular UPF. Framing prepared foods that way makes it much easier to walk past them without buying. Over time, that mantra has become ingrained. My perception of the boxes of sugary cereals has changed

203

drastically because of my mindset. I wouldn't buy them, but more importantly, I'm not tempted to buy them.

Reframing fasting and snacking

For many people, fasting carries many negative connotations. A lot of us have grown up believing that snacks are healthy and fasting is unhealthy. For most people, the exact opposite is true. Fasting is simply a time that you allow your body to use the calories it has stored (as sugar or body fat). Snacks change your body from a fasted (calorie-burning) state to a fed (calorie-storing) state.

Here are some common automatic thoughts around snacking and fasting:

- Snacks are healthy.
- I should eat multiple snacks a day.
- Fasting is unhealthy.
- Fasting is hard.
- Never skip breakfast.

Replace these automatic thoughts by deliberately saying to yourself:
- Snacks are an occasional indulgence.
- Snacks are just extra calories.
- Fasting is just taking a break from eating.
- Fasting allows the body to "eat its own fat."
- Fasting cleanses the body.
- Fasting allows the body to purify itself.

We want to reframe fasting as inherently beneficial to the body and as a practice that anybody can do. At the same time, we want to reframe snacking as an occasional indulgence and nothing more.

Come up with a personal "reframing mantra" that will help reprogram negative associations with positive ones. During fasting, my personal mantra to help deal with hunger is to think to myself, "Burn, baby, burn," as I rub my stomach. I am reminded that my body is burning the dangerous visceral fat, and that thought helps me see hunger as a sign of progress.

What's on your mind matters more than what's on your plate. It's not about willpower. It's not simply a matter of knowing what diet to follow—Mediterranean, low fat, low carb, keto, vegan, or another. Success comes only when you also master the emotional, the social, and the societal side of weight loss. That all starts with your mindset. The next step is to ingrain healthy habits.

CULTIVATING HEALTHY SOCIAL EATING HABITS

ESTABLISHED HABITS DO NOT require thought or willpower to implement. Take brushing your teeth, for example. Do you ever think consciously about doing it anymore? Probably not. Brushing your teeth has become a habit—yet the dividends of good dental hygiene continue.

You can establish a new habit in about two to three weeks, and the payoff can provide a lifetime of benefits. If you are in the habit of walking to work every day, you will receive the daily benefits without willpower or effort. For example, the average resident of Tokyo walks 8611 steps daily, which is almost 4 miles (nearly 6.5 km)![1] They don't think about walking, or even barely notice they're doing it, but the benefits accrue day after day. The secret power of the healthy habit, like brushing your teeth or walking, is that it makes positive benefits automatic.

Habits work against you as well. If you habitually eat late-night snacks or binge in front of the television, you'll get hungry every time you find yourself in that situation. Habits are self-perpetuating, because the longer the habit persists, the more established it becomes. If you are overeating because of your habits, then you need to change those habits, not "just Eat Less."

When establishing new eating habits, keep each change clear and simple, because complexity is the enemy of execution. Here are some examples:

- Eat only two meals per day.
- Eat satiating foods at mealtimes. Avoid eating between meals.
- Eat only in designated areas.
- Eat natural foods. Avoid ultra-processed foods.
- Don't eat all the time.
- Fast for sixteen hours a day every day, except for Saturday.
- Fast for the first five days of every month.
- Eat mindfully.
- Walk after each meal.
- Don't eat "naked" carbs.
- Eat leafy green vegetables with every meal.

Simple. Clear. Obvious. Each statement can be groomed into an actionable habit that can pay dividends for life. You can stack your habits (eating two meals a day, fasting sixteen hours a day, eating only natural foods at a table) to set your body fat thermostat for automatic weight loss. Think of these habits as your personal food "rules" that you follow automatically and without question. Committing to your rules eliminates the "Should I or shouldn't I?" question in your mind.

Compare this advice to cultivate a new healthy eating habit to the "gold standard" weight-loss advice of "Eat 500 fewer calories per day" of whatever foods you want whenever and wherever you want. Consider the complexity of this hare-brained scheme. With the standard weight-loss advice:

- you have no simple, easy-to-follow rules, since all foods have different calories;
- you don't cultivate a healthy mindset for weight loss;
- you establish no healthy habits;
- you have no default to a healthy eating pattern. In fact, you get no guidance whatsoever;
- you don't get help addressing ultra-processed foods, food addiction, or emotional eating;

- you don't get help addressing the social or societal aspects of eating behavior; and
- you judge foods purely by their caloric content, without regard for their level of processing, speed of digestion and absorption, food matrix, order of eating, and so on.

Standard weight-loss advice provides no structure on which to build a successful system to maintain a healthy weight. Standard weight-loss advice establishes no healthy eating habits. Bad habits are allowed to fester like unruptured pustules on your face.

> **Tip #49:** Cultivate a health mindset
> to make healthy eating a habit.

How to break bad habits

Sometimes you might have to break bad habits before you create new and healthier ones. Use a five-step approach (Figure 12.2).

Figure 12.2. How to break a bad habit in five steps

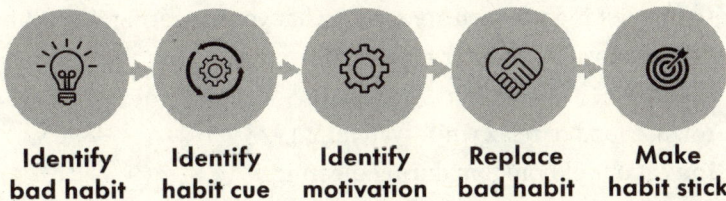

| Identify | Identify | Identify | Replace | Make |
| bad habit | habit cue | motivation | bad habit | habit stick |

First, identify the bad habits and then try to neutralize them. Going "cold turkey" on bad habits is not always the most effective strategy. Instead, it is often easier and more effective to swap a problematic habit with a healthier one.

207

Step 1: Identify the problematic habit
Examples:
- Snacking
- Using food as a reward
- Eating until overly full
- Eating in your car, picking up food at the drive-thru
- Eating mindlessly while watching TV or spectator events
- Eating out of boredom
- Eating whatever is available or offered

Step 2: Identify the cue to the bad habit
Cues are triggers or reminders to engage in a habit. Buying a coffee may be the cue to buy a muffin or donut. Watching TV may be a cue to eat potato chips.
Examples:
- Coffee breaks
- Work meetings
- Watching TV or movies
- Long car rides

Step 3: Identify the motivation for the habit
Try to understand why you are eating what you are eating. Think about the "three whys" of Chapter 1 (page 20).
Examples:
- You use food to relax while watching TV.
- You eat out of boredom during meetings.
- You eat because you feel sad or lonely.

Step 4: Replace the bad habit with a healthy one
208 Make sure your new habit supports your healthy eating goals.
Examples:
- Drink sparkling water or tea instead of soda, alcohol, or juice.
- Celebrate your successes with something other than food—a massage, a new pair of shoes, a pedicure, a collectible.

- Plate your meal and eat mindfully, putting down your fork between bites.
- While watching TV, occupy your hands with crafts like knitting.
- Do something active when you're bored—talk to a friend, go for a walk, do a jigsaw puzzle.

Step 5: Make your healthy habit stick

Think about strategies to help you choose your healthy new habit.
   Examples:
- Use a habit tracker so you can see your progress.
- Keep green tea easily available in your kitchen.
- Think ahead and make sure you have the supplies for your new habit on hand.
- Make the cues for your new healthy habit visible—keep your crochet set beside the TV, leave your jigsaw puzzles out on the table or a shelf, peel and cut carrot or celery sticks and put them in the fridge so that they are easily available to add to your lunch bag or dinner plate.

How to create new habits

Once you've broken or switched the bad habits, it's time to create new healthy habits that can help you maintain your weight loss. Use a similar five-step process (Figure 12.3).

Figure 12.3. How to create a healthy new habit in five steps

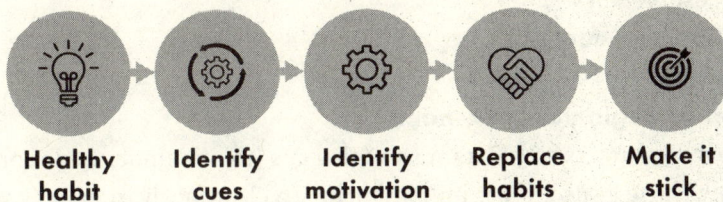

| Healthy habit | Identify cues | Identify motivation | Replace habits | Make it stick |

Step 1: Identify a new healthy habit you'd like to incorporate

You can set SMART (specific, measurable, achievable, relevant, and time-bound) goals.

Examples:

- Drinking eight glasses water daily, instead of sugary/sweet drinks
- Walking for at least thirty minutes after dinner daily
- Practicing positive self-talk about fasting and eating healthy daily
- Eating mindfully using your personal mantra at least once a day, remembering to eat slowly and only until 80 percent full (page 143)
- Following a regular fasting plan—time-restricted eating (fasting for eighteen of twenty-four hours), or fasting for twenty-four, thirty-six, or forty-two hours

Step 2: Identify the cues you can use to engage in the healthy habit

Cues are triggers or reminders to engage in a habit. Brewing a large pot of green tea at breakfast may be the cue to drink more tea throughout the day.

Examples:

- Set up three 24 oz (~700 mL) bottles of water to start the day so you drink more water.
- Leave your walking shoes out where you can easily see them.
- Write "hara hachi bu" on a note and leave it on your dining table.

Step 3: Identify the motivation for your new habit

Try to understand why you want to create this habit.

Examples:

- Lower your blood glucose levels
- Lose weight
- Improve your health

Step 4: Begin your new habit

The most successful habits start with a cue (the reminder to do something), have a specific action, and include a clear motivation (why you want to do it). Write down the cue, habit, and motivation for your habit.

Examples:

- Every Monday (cue), I will skip breakfast and lunch and eat a small dinner (habit), to lose the weekend weight (motivation).

- Every meal (cue), I will drink green tea (habit) so that I am not tempted by sugary drinks or alcoholic drinks, to keep my blood glucose down (motivation).
- On Sunday and Wednesday (cue) before I eat dinner, I will prep one meal for the week or the freezer (habit), to make sticking to my diet easier (motivation).

Step 5: Make your healthy habit stick
Think about strategies to help you choose your healthy new habit.
- Use your habit tracker.
- Write down your habit and pin it to the refrigerator door. Write down your habit and make it your smartphone's wallpaper.
- Tell a partner/spouse/coach about your new habit to stay accountable (see below).
- Make achieving your habit a game. Every time you follow the habit, give yourself ten points, and reward yourself when you reach 100 points with a massage, collectible, or pedicure.

Learn from others
Thinking about "naturally" skinny people who seem to eat whatever they want and still stay thin may make you want to pull out your hair. However, learning what habits they have in common can be a useful exercise in forming new healthy habits of your own. Here are a few examples.

1. **They are busy living life.** Lean people always seem to be busy—at work, school, volunteering, helping others, playing tennis, walking, working out, fishing. These active hobbies largely preclude eating, as opposed to watching movies or TV or pleasure cruising. These people are never eating out of boredom because they're always doing something active.
2. **They eat slowly and mindfully.** Many lean people enjoy food a lot, and they are constantly trying out new recipes and new restaurants. My aunt and uncle, for example, love food; they have an "eating club"

where they meet friends to try different restaurants around the city. They are super-skinny, with a body mass index of less than 22. Their secret? When they eat, they savor each bite for what seems like forever. They invariably don't eat a lot, but they always feel very full.

3. **They don't finish all the food on their plate.** When lean people are full, they stop eating. At restaurants, they pack the leftovers, even a single bite. They feel no compulsion to "clean their plate." Why eat food that you are not enjoying and that makes you gain weight that you'll struggle to lose? It's a lose-lose situation. I once ordered a dessert with a friend. It wasn't good, so I pushed it away. My friend was slightly shocked, saying that I shouldn't waste it. I was shocked in turn. The dessert was full of sugar, the money was already spent, and it wasn't healthy. If I wasn't enjoying it, then why would I eat it?

4. **They don't turn to food in times of emotional distress or out of habit.** Lean people will tend to talk to a friend, go for a walk, or take a long bath to help process their emotions. And their default setting is to be active rather than eating.

Once you've mastered your mindset, broken your bad habits, and replaced them with good ones, it's time to make sure you stay on track by using the social power of your group.

Adding accountability

Humans are social creatures, so almost everything is easier when you do with it with a friend. This fact is also true for weight loss.[2] Peer pressure can compel kids to do outrageous things. That is the power of the social group and social influence, mostly with a negative connotation. As adults, this same power can be harnessed to create lasting positive change. Peer **support**—whether it is Weight Watchers or Alcoholics Anonymous or a running club or a reading group or a knitting club or an online fasting community—makes what seems difficult or impossible a routine.

Groups are powerful motivators because they force us to be accountable to others. And the group's expectations that we will do what we say we'll do makes us feel obliged to do it. For example, I play tennis every Monday, so I show up every week, even when I'm not particularly motivated. I know that others will notice if I skip that week.

When I do a longer fast, I tell my family, which helps to keep me accountable. Otherwise, I might be tempted to simply skip it. By adding an extra accountability step, my dropout rate is close to 0 percent, because if I don't fast, I will look foolish.

I co-founded an online fasting community at The Fasting Method (TheFastingMethod.com) to help people stick to their fasting and weight-loss goals, while providing useful advice and guidance. The results have been impressive: many members have lost over 100 pounds (45 kg). Several have been so successful, they've changed their careers to coach others in their weight-loss journey.

While our online community provides knowledge, that is not the main purpose. The true benefit is to normalize fasting, create lasting habits, and provide social models for success. If everybody around you is fasting, you will be more likely to follow. The Fasting Method provides personalized and small-group coaching for weight loss, which I've always thought was underutilized as an accountability tool. When people want to get in shape, they get a personal trainer, not because they can't google an exercise program, but because they need the extra accountability and expertise that comes with hiring a professional. Adding a personal coach can be the difference between achieving your goals and not.

> **Tip #50:** Find a weight-loss buddy or join a weight-loss group.

THE THIRD GOLDEN RULE: COMMIT TO A HEALTH MINDSET AND HEALTHY SOCIAL HABITS

The social habits that we form, and the people we surround ourselves with, are one of the most important factors in weight gain. If you lived in 1970s America, you were highly unlikely to have obesity. If you live in America today, you are highly likely to have obesity, because the U.S. is an obesogenic environment. Your weight gain is not your fault, because it is the product of the environment in which you live. Almost every aspect of eating is affected by where we live and who we know.

Social habits influence everything about eating behavior, from what we eat to how much we eat, where we eat, when we eat, and how we eat. Creating a social network for sustained weight loss, including the proper mindset and habits, is a lot of work. But, hey, welcome to the real world. While the headline on the supermarket tabloid screams "Do This One Thing and Lose Weight Forever!," we all know it isn't true. Obesity is a multifactorial disease. You might be able to lose weight for a while doing that one thing, but to sustain the weight loss? Long-term weight loss requires a change in mindset, habits, and actions.

Once you've laid the foundation with my three Golden Rules, you can create a durable structure to scaffold your weight-loss plan.

| 13 |

PUTTING THE
GOLDEN RULES OF WEIGHT
LOSS INTO ACTION

T HE MOST INTOXICATING part of most weight-loss shows is the before-and-after reveal, or the "aha" moment when people jump onstage in their moment of triumph. On live television in 1988, talk show host Oprah Winfrey, wearing skinny jeans, famously walked onstage pulling a little red wagon filled with 67 pounds (30 kg) of animal fat that represented the weight she'd lost following a strict calorie-restricted diet. She proudly told her studio audience: "If you can believe in yourself...you can conquer it."

The underlying premise of Oprah's statement and most others is "Just eat fewer calories" and you too can be an inspiring weight-loss winner in life! This type of pronouncement is usually entwined with some hopeful and thin-spirational nonsense about willpower. "You just have to want it enough." "If you can dream it, you can do it." Did this approach work long term for Oprah? Well, no.

Looking back in 2005, Oprah wrote: "What I didn't know [in 1988] was that my metabolism was shot. Two weeks after returning to real food, I was up 10 pounds...Seventeen years after that show, I know a whole lot better."[1] What was it that she should have known? A calorie is not a calorie. The standard "expert" advice focused only on calories is guaranteed to fail. People who diet desperately count their calories like Ebenezer Scrooge counted his pennies, yet almost all ultimately fail. The problem was never the calories. The problem was never the willpower. The problem is the hunger—homeostatic, hedonic, and conditioned. "Calories" is a single factor in a multifactorial disease, and likely one of the least important.

To the person with a hammer, every problem is a nail. In other words, you can't solve a problem until you find its root cause.

THE ROOT CAUSE OF OBESITY IS MORE COMPLEX THAN CALORIES

IN MEDICINE, a symptom *indicates* an underlying disease but is not the disease itself. For example, a fever is a symptom that may be caused by various diseases or disease agents like viruses, bacteria, cancer, autoimmune diseases, and so on. Treating the symptom, just like taking a pill like acetaminophen or aspirin, doesn't treat the disease. A fundamental principle of medicine is to treat the disease, not the symptom. For a fever, for example, you may need an antiviral, antibiotic, chemotherapy, or anti-inflammatory medication. This standard rigorous approach to treating disease seems have completely eluded obesity medicine.

Weight gain is a symptom of an underlying problem but not the problem itself. You must find the root cause and address it (Table 13.1). Weight gain has many potential root causes and, therefore, many potential treatments. If your weight problem is caused by food addiction, then eating fewer calories won't help. If your weight problem is mindless or distracted eating, then eating fewer calories won't help. If your weight gain is caused by lack of sleep, then eating fewer calories won't help.

216

Table 13.1. Some of the many root causes of weight gain and what to do about them

Symptom	Root cause	Solution	Typical "expert" solution
Weight gain	Refined carbs	Fewer carbs	It's all about calories. Eat less.
Weight gain	High Glycemic Index carbs	Slower carbs	It's all about calories. Eat less.
Weight gain	No fiber	More fiber	It's all about calories. Eat less.
Weight gain	Food matrix	Whole foods	It's all about calories. Eat less.
Weight gain	Naked carbs	Mixed meals	It's all about calories. Eat less.
Weight gain	Eating late	Eating earlier	It's all about calories. Eat less.
Weight gain	UPFs	Whole foods	It's all about calories. Eat less.
Weight gain	Sugary drinks	Water, tea, coffee	It's all about calories. Eat less.
Weight gain	Food addiction	Counseling	It's all about calories. Eat less.
Weight gain	Distracted eating	Mindful eating	It's all about calories. Eat less.
Weight gain	Eating too often	Fasting more	It's all about calories. Eat less.
Weight gain	Eating too fast	Eating slowly	It's all about calories. Eat less.
Weight gain	Expectation effect	Avoiding "diet" foods	It's all about calories. Eat less.

Symptom	Root cause	Solution	Typical "expert" solution
Weight gain	Hunger cues	Avoiding cues	It's all about calories. Eat less.
Weight gain	Poor sleep	Improving sleep	It's all about calories. Eat less.
Weight gain	Boredom	Getting a hobby	It's all about calories. Eat less.
Weight gain	Mindless eating	Structured eating	It's all about calories. Eat less.
Weight gain	Emotional eating	Peer support	It's all about calories. Eat less.
Weight gain	Poor habits	Habit change	It's all about calories. Eat less.
Weight gain	Social modeling	Peer support	It's all about calories. Eat less.
Weight gain	Too much sugar	Less sugar	It's all about calories. Eat less.
Weight gain	Depression	Psychotherapy	It's all about calories. Eat less.
Weight gain	Chronic stress	Meditation	It's all about calories. Eat less.

While all these possible root causes and solutions may seem complicated, that's real life. The alternative is to accept that weight loss is as simple as Calories In, Calories Out and doom yourself to a lifetime of tears.

No single treatment, summarized by that hideous term "energy balance" can possibly be the solution to every problem that causes obesity. And guess what? It isn't, despite so many protestations to "cut calories" (and hit fewer icebergs).

You would be (rightly) skeptical if I told you there is a single treatment that cures all cancers. You would be (rightly) skeptical if I said there is a single drug that cures all infections. You'd be (rightly) skeptical if I said there is a single cure for all genetic diseases. But when a single treatment (calorie restriction) is proclaimed to cure all the causes of weight gain, "experts" call it the most scientifically accurate advice ever known. Let me say it again: "overeating" is really an "over-hunger" problem, which covers all of the broad topics of homeostatic, hedonic, and conditioned hunger. Calories are a component but not the whole of homeostatic, or physiological, hunger. Calories have nothing to do with emotional or social hunger, which are equally—if not sometimes more—important root causes of weight gain. This is strange, because calories don't even exist in human physiology.

THE GOLDEN RULES OF WEIGHT LOSS

JAMES CLEAR, AUTHOR of *Atomic Habits*, says: "You do not rise to the level of your goals. You fall to the level of your systems."[2] Having a goal, such as winning a sports championship, is largely meaningless. Both winners and losers have the same goal. What distinguishes winners and losers are the systems they put in place to achieve those goals. What is the plan for recruitment, training, fitness, strategy, teamwork, nutrition, and so on?

Similarly, the goals to "lose weight" or even simply "eat less" are, by themselves, meaningless. The point is to create a system that leads you to success and includes effective strategies that must address

1. **knowledge** (homeostatic hunger),
2. **emotions** (hedonic hunger), and
3. **environments** (conditioned hunger).

The most important factors of homeostatic hunger are the hormones that govern the body's fat thermostat—insulin, leptin, GLP-1, peptide YY, and so on—and how things like nutrients and the food matrix and gastric emptying may affect them. But knowledge is, by itself, not enough to create lasting change.

Just because you know that cookies are fattening doesn't mean you won't eat them. Just because you know you should switch your french fries for a side salad doesn't mean you will. Just because you know that exercising is good for you doesn't mean that you'll do it. If only life were that simple.

After gaining the proper knowledge, you must control the emotional component of weight loss. We eat the cookies because they give us pleasure and make us feel better (temporarily). That is reality. How can we address these emotional triggers to tame hedonic hunger? Understanding ultra-processed foods, food addictions, and emotional eating is a start.

Perhaps the most important factors of all are societal and social factors. We succeed when our friends and family who surround us succeed. We succeed when societal norms allow healthy eating behaviors to be the easy choice. It is effortless to not eat cookies during an afternoon meeting if none are readily available. It is hard to not eat cookies if they are sitting in front of us. It is easy to avoid late-night snacking if no snacks are around.

Successful weight loss as a goal is much, much more than managing calories. You must also

- manage hunger and satiety,
- manage food addictions and cravings,
- manage emotions,
- manage mindless and distracted eating,
- manage habits,
- manage deprivation mindset,
- manage your food environment, and
- manage holiday and vacation eating.

Yes, successful weight loss means thinking about many factors. However, these factors boil down to three key actions that address many of the root causes of homeostatic, hedonic, and conditioned hunger.

These are the three Golden Rules of weight loss:

1. Avoid ultra-processed foods.
2. Don't eat all the time. Fast regularly.
3. Develop the proper mindsets and social habits.

The first Golden Rule: Avoid ultra-processed foods

In *The Obesity Code*, I suggested avoiding added sugars and refined carbohydrates, eating a moderate amount of protein, and not fearing natural dietary fats. Avoiding ultra-processed foods is a simple way to avoid most of those worst offenders. Many UPFs are very high in added sugars, refined carbohydrates, and refined fats and also low in protein and natural fats. Furthermore, the refining process affects the food matrix, speed of digestion, and speed of absorption, causing massive spikes in glucose and insulin. Hunger is maximized and satiety is minimized. Chemicals are added to make the food very rewarding, often with huge dopamine spikes. UPFs are almost perfectly designed to make you gain weight. The heavy advertising and endorsements used by UPF brands create a social environment and culture where eating them constantly feels normal.

Does this first Golden Rule reduce

- homeostatic hunger? Yes.
- hedonic hunger? Yes.
- conditioned hunger? Yes.

221

The second Golden Rule:
Don't eat all the time. Fast regularly.

In *The Obesity Code*, I also suggested adding regular fasting, which effectively allows insulin levels to fall. Fasting switches our bodies from fat-storing mode to fat-burning mode. Fasting regularly is still great advice, and in the time since that book was published, both the lay public and the research community have taken an interest in intermittent fasting. In addition to its effect on reducing insulin levels, fasting helps reduce hunger (long term), due to its ghrelin and sympathetic nervous system effects, and to reduce UPF consumption, and the abstinence feature of fasting helps break food addictions and emotional eating. Fasting also rebuilds structure into the eating day and reinforces healthy eating habits.

Fasting may have even more benefits than weight loss: helping to break down and recycle damaged cells (autophagy), decrease inflammation, and prevent disease, and allowing us to live longer. These topics are covered more thoroughly in my book *The Complete Guide to Fasting*.

Does this second Golden Rule reduce

- homeostatic hunger? Yes.
- hedonic hunger? Yes.
- conditioned hunger? Yes.

The third Golden Rule:
Commit to a health mindset and healthy social habits

The third, and arguably the most important aspect of weight loss, is to create a lasting social system that allows you to maintain success. Manage your mindset and create social circles that support weight loss, deal with addictions and emotions, break the bad habits, and create new healthier habits. All these actions underlie behavior change, which is ultimately the only way to lose weight and keep it off. Peer support is a critical aspect of all human endeavors, and weight loss is no exception.

Habitually eating fewer meals per day makes you hungry less often. Habitually eating smaller meals makes you less hungry overall.

Having peer support means you rely less on ultra-processed foods to "self-medicate" your anxiety or depression, and you have many people to model healthy eating habits.

Does this this third Golden Rule help reduce

- homeostatic hunger? Yes.
- hedonic hunger? Yes.
- conditioned hunger? Yes.

The simplistic advice to "Eat fewer calories" doesn't adequately address any of these three dimensions of successful behavior change: knowledge, emotions, and social/environmental factors. None of the most important factors of weight loss are low willpower or self-control.

FOLLOWING THE TRIED AND TRUE
AND SUBTRACTING FOR SIMPLICITY

THE EXTRAORDINARY THINKER and writer Nassim Nicholas Taleb, author of *Antifragile* and *Skin in the Game*, describes a theory of survivability he calls the Lindy Effect. The idea is that the longer something nonperishable has been in existence, the longer it is likely to continue existing. For example, books, songs, and ideas closely follow this heuristic. Shakespeare's play *A Midsummer Night's Dream* was published circa 1595 and will likely continue being published. The song "Happy Birthday to You" was probably first published in 1924 and will likely continue in popularity. The classic movie *The Sound of Music* was first released in 1965 and will likely continue to be watched. Simply put, an idea or tradition that has stuck around for a long time probably has a lot of value.

The Lindy Effect also applies to traditional food advice. For example, if your mother, grandmother, and great-grandmother follow certain food rules, then it's likely that advice will continue to be good. Avoiding fake, artificial foods—now called ultra-processed foods—and eating traditional, ancestral, natural foods is probably one of the oldest food rules in existence. In its zeal to equate all foods to their caloric content,

223

the "religion" of Calories In, Calories Out temporarily sidelined this idea. For a time, people believed that eating ultra-processed foods that were low in fat was very healthy.

Similarly, the Lindy Effect applies to fasting. Fasting, too, is likely one of the oldest food rules in existence. This practice has been part of human history for thousands of years and will likely continue to be. People do not fast for fun. Traditionally, they deliberately avoided eating all the time to improve their overall health. The idea that we should constantly eat, or "graze," didn't even last a few decades.

The idea of creating socially supportive groups with like-minded goals and habits, such as with organized religions and churches, has been around for thousands of years and will likely continue for thousands of years.

Time acts as a filter. Ideas that survive for generations have proven their robustness. In the internet age, people often chase the latest, greatest fad diet. These Golden Rules for weight loss are not that. They are ancient ideas that have withstood the test of time. Therein lies their power.

Taleb also describes the idea of Via Negativa, or adding by subtracting. Amateurs focus on what to do. Professionals focus on what to *not* do. They focus on taking away, not adding. Removing what is wrong, harmful, or unnecessary increases simplicity, and thereby effectiveness. A good golfer focuses on how to hit the ball. A great golfer focuses on removing all extraneous movements except for hitting that ball. The first two Golden Rules of weight loss focus on Via Negativa. Do *not* eat UPFs. Do *not* eat all the time.

A DIETARY PLAN FOR LOSING WEIGHT AUTOMATICALLY

A DIETARY PLAN that focuses exclusively on a single lonely factor such as calories fails virtually every time. A successful dietary plan is anchored by addressing all the questions of weight loss: **who, what, when, where, why, and how**.

Who to eat with:
Eat with people who share your weight-loss goals

Try to always eat with somebody who shares your ideals and weight-loss goals. If you eat regularly with somebody who has poor eating habits, those poor habits will rub off on you. If you eat regularly with somebody who has healthy eating habits, those healthy habits will rub off on you. But here's the thing. *You* get to decide who you eat with. The presence of a friend or family adds accountability, a key component of cultivating social habits.

Whenever I eat with my family, I eat a lot more non-starchy vegetables and a lot fewer french fries. When I eat with my high school friends, I eat a lot more junk food and sugary drinks. Who I eat with determines what I eat, how much I eat, how fast I eat, and so on. That very fact makes *who* a very important question to ask.

What to eat: A low-insulin diet

Eat a low-insulin diet that maximizes the satiety hormones to fill you up and keep you full. Eat enough less-fattening foods (lots of healthy natural fats, moderate amounts of protein) so that you'll be less tempted to eat the more-fattening foods (refined carbohydrates) later on. For example, you don't want to "cut calories" by eating less grilled chicken and salad at lunch, because you'll be more tempted to eat cookies in the mid-afternoon. It's just like Mom used to say if you asked for a bedtime snack: "You should have eaten more at dinner."

Include the following foods in your diet:

- Meats and poultry: beef, lamb, pork, chicken
- Fish (cod, halibut, salmon, tuna, sardines) and seafood (shrimp, crab, oysters, mussels, clams)
- Dairy: eggs, cheeses (all kinds—cheddar, halloumi, feta, ricotta, mozzarella, brie, cottage cheese), full-fat yogurt, butter, Greek yogurt
- Nuts and seeds: pumpkin, sunflower, almonds, Brazil nuts, hazelnuts, walnuts, macadamia, chia, flax, pumpkin, hemp. Be careful about peanuts, cashews, and pistachios, which are higher in carbohydrates.

225

- Vegetables: mushrooms, cauliflower, broccoli, zucchini, leafy greens (lettuce, kale, spinach), asparagus, artichokes, bok choy, carrots, onions, tomatoes, cucumber, beans
- Pulses and legumes: lentils, quinoa, tofu
- Acidic and fermented foods: pickles, vinegar, lemon juice, sauerkraut, kimchi, tempeh
- Fruits: avocados, olives, berries
- Fats: olive oil, avocado oil, coconut oil, lard, beef tallow
- Spices: pepper, chili, garlic, ginger, turmeric, rosemary, cinnamon, cardamom

What not to eat

Avoid ultra-processed foods. They can make you hungrier and are often sold as healthy foods, but they're not. Avoid insulin-spiking foods.

Here are some popular "healthy" foods that really are not healthy at all:

- Processed fruits: fruit yogurt, dried fruit, fruit juice, canned fruit, agave nectar
- Sugary fruits: watermelon, grapes, pineapple, papaya
- Granola, protein/fiber bars
- Diet sodas
- "Low-fat" foods: fat-free commercial salad dressings, fat-free yogurt
- "Low-fat" snacks: crackers, baked chips, pita chips
- Low-calorie sweeteners
- Commercial peanut butter
- Processed cheese
- Processed meats, lunch meats
- Plant-based meats
- Processed oils, vegetable oils, palm oil, hydrogenated oils, margarine
- Oat milk, rice milk

BEWARE PROCESSED "HEALTH" FOODS

The label "plant-based" is meant to convey that a food is automatically healthy, but plant-based meats are a fake food that goes way, way beyond regular ultra-processed food. These "meats" are mega-processed chemistry experiments. No naturally occurring soybean, pea, or mushroom tastes like meat, has the texture of meat, smells like meat, or looks like meat. Changing plant-based proteins into something that resembles meat takes a whole battery of substances concocted in a chemist's lab. Healthy? Hardly.

Take "vegan chicken nuggets" or "vegan bacon," for example. These products often start with a low-cost industrial-grade protein, say an animal-grade soy protein. That "plant base" is mixed with highly processed vegetable oil, industrial-grade fillers, artificial flavors and colors, chemical texturizers, and other additives. The "meat" is then coated in preservatives to keep it "fresh."

When you eat plants (vegetables), make sure they're easily recognizable as plants (vegetables). For example, great substitutes for meat include dried beans, mushrooms, eggplant (think eggplant parm), and chickpeas. Tofu is also a good substitute.

"Vegan" milks, like oat and rice milk, are another example of a highly processed "health" food. These "milks" are basically just starch juice that spikes blood glucose. The Glycemic Index of oat milk is high at 60 compared to 37 for dairy milk and nut milks. Oat milk contains the sugar maltose, which is two glucose molecules stuck together. Rice milk has a staggeringly high Glycemic Index of 85 to 90. Instead of oat and rice milks, consider soy or nut milks, although concerns have been raised about phytoestrogens in soy and environmental degradation caused by making nut milks.

227

Salad is a healthy choice, but commercial salad dressings usually are not. They often contain processed vegetable oils, added sugars, and artificial flavors. For example, a nationally available commercial creamy Caesar dressing contains the following ingredients: water, vegetable oil, sugars, Parmesan cheese, vinegar, liquid yolk, salt, seasoning, modified cornstarch, garlic, lactic acid, sorbic acid, xanthan gum, polysorbate 60, yeast extract, caramel, calcium disodium EDTA, paprika oleoresin, and turmeric oleoresin. What should be a healthy salad becomes a bowl full of sugar and unpronounceable ingredients. Instead of buying commercial salad dressings, make your own using olive oil, lemon juice or vinegar, plus whatever herbs or spices you like.

To add flavor to your salad and keep you full, add some protein. Try grilled fish, chicken, or beef, or beans, tofu, or nuts.

What to drink

Don't drink your calories. Thick fluids like soups increase satiety and feel more like a meal.

- **Do** drink plenty of water, sparkling water, tea, herbal tea, and coffee so that you're not so thirsty.
- **Do not** drink juices, sodas, and alcohol.

When to eat: Eat early—and only when you're hungry

Set a specific time to eat, whether that meal is once, twice, or three times per day. This schedule creates a scaffold for your weight-loss plan. Eating earlier is better than eating later but balance this ideal timing against the social realities of your life.

Brush your teeth after dinner as a reminder that you shouldn't eat. Adding a small disincentive, like knowing that you'll have to brush your teeth again if you wind up snacking, can help to curb the habit.

When you schedule your meals, you make sure that your body gets time to fast. Fasting is a time-honored method of letting your body "eat" its stored calories (your body fat). The standard fasting period for everybody should be twelve to fourteen hours almost every day, which simply means eating dinner at 7 p.m. and breakfast by 7 to 9 a.m. If you want to increase the fasting period, consult with your health care provider first if you have medical concerns. Then you can try fasts of sixteen, eighteen, twenty-four, or thirty-six hours or more knowing that you have the support of your doctor. At TheFastingMethod.com, members often use a five-day modified fast monthly to reset.

Remember that time is not running out. There is always time for another fast.

Where to eat: Eat at a table

Eat only at places designated for eating, such as a dining or kitchen table or a cafeteria. This strategy will help you stick to your structured weight-loss plan. If you cannot eat at that designated spot, then simply don't eat.

Why eat?

You might eat because you are hungry, but more likely you eat because it is time to eat. Before you prep or sit down for a meal, understand why you are eating. Be mindful: is your hunger homeostatic (physiological), hedonic (emotional), or conditioned (socially influenced)? Once you know, you can make the necessary adjustments.

How much to eat: Eat until you are 80 percent full

What you eat determines **how much** you eat. Some foods are filling. Some foods are not filling. Some foods make you hungrier. Some foods do not. Know the difference, which is based on our body's hormonal response, not calories. Don't eat foods that make you hungrier.

And don't count your calories. Eat until you are nearly full (hara hachi bu).

229

CONCLUDING THOUGHTS

MY GOAL IN writing *The Obesity Code* and this follow-up, *The Hunger Code,* is to describe the intricate and nuanced science of weight gain and weight loss and the underlying factors that have precipitated our obesity epidemic.

For one person, eating less white bread may be the key to losing weight. But for another person, dealing with emotional trauma may be the key to keeping that weight off. For a third person, weight loss may mean cutting out the sugar that they use to self-medicate their depression. No one solution is universally right or wrong. Each solution addresses a different root cause, and the root cause of obesity can be different for different people.

The Diet Wars continue because one person insists that the solution to weight gain is all about eating less white bread, a second insists it's all about trauma counseling, and a third insists it's all about cutting out sugar. Each person insists that the others are incorrect because we've all been told for decades that weight gain can only be about one single thing. No medical disease works like that, and obesity is a disease. The belief that weight gain is about one thing (calories) is as silly as arguing that a fever is only caused by a virus, or a bacterium, or an inflammatory disease, or an allergy. Each person can be correct, as long as they understand the multifactorial nature of the disease (the obesity or the fever).

Weight gain is only a symptom that may be triggered by many different root causes.

In the end, the deeper understanding of the root causes of obesity helps us to treat each other with empathy and compassion. When you know better, you can do better. *The Hunger Code* is a continuation of *The Obesity Code,* so I'll reiterate: a new hope arises.

WEIGHT-LOSS TIPS

Tip #1: Don't count calories.

Tip #2: Understand that foods contain both calories and information about what to do with those calories.

Tip #3: Exercise for its many health benefits, but not for weight loss.

Tip #4: Focus on the neurohormonal factors to lose weight. Obesity is a hormonal rather than a caloric imbalance and different foods affect hormones differently.

Tip #5: Eat fewer refined (starchy) carbohydrates.

Tip #6: Choose foods with a low Glycemic Index and glycemic load and avoid rapidly digested starches.

Tip #7: Keep carbohydrates as natural and unprocessed as possible. Prefer coarsely ground (stone-ground) rather than finely ground (machine-ground) flour due to its larger particle size.

Tip #8: Choose amylose starches like quinoa, lentils, baby potatoes, oats, and beans.

Tip #9: Eat more fiber to satisfy hunger and keep insulin low.

Tip #10: Eat steel cut oats, not instant, for their high-soluble fiber.

Tip #11: Eat more resistant starches. Cook, cool, and reheat rice. Eat cooked potatoes cold.

Tip #12: Choose pasta and low-glycemic rice over white bread.

Tip #13: Eat whole fruits, not cooked, puréed, or juiced fruits.

Tip #14: Blend seeded fruits into smoothies to release their fiber and other nutrients.

Tip #15: Choose lower-fructose fruits like berries and avoid higher-fructose fruits like grapes, mangoes, and watermelon.

Tip #16: Drink thicker, slower-digesting liquids like soup. Add chia seeds for viscosity and fiber.

Tip #17: Eat more acidic foods, including vinegar (pickled foods), fermented foods (sauerkraut, kimchi), and lemon juice.

Tip #18: Always eat your carbs with proteins and fats. Don't eat "naked" carbs.

Tip #19: Eat carbohydrates last in your meal.

Tip #20: Eat meals earlier in the day, especially meals containing carbs. Avoid large, late dinners and snacks.

Tip #21: Eat bulky, heavy foods that contain fiber and water to fill the stomach, such as leafy green vegetables, berries, beans, whole oats, cauliflower, and broccoli.

Tip #22: Increase both duration and quality of sleep.

Tip #23: Use moderate exercise to temporarily control hunger.

Tip #24: Don't fear natural fats, but don't eat more than necessary. Avoid foods labeled "low fat" or "fat free."

Tip #25: Prioritize a moderate amount of protein for its neuro-hormonal satiety effects (GLP-1, PYY, and CCK).

Tip #26: Eat naturally protein-rich foods, not ultra-processed protein powders.

Tip #27: Eat more bitter foods, including turmeric.

Tip #28: Drink lots of green, oolong, and black tea.

Tip #29: Drink more coffee.

Tip #30: Avoid "diet" sodas and "sugar-free" foods.

Tip #31: Learn to recognize signs of food addiction, abstain from ultra-processed foods, and seek support.

Tip #32: Avoid distracted eating. Eat only at a table in a designated place—kitchen, dining room—and turn off or put away tech devices.

Tip #33: Enhance your memory of food by choosing highly seasoned, spicy, and high-umami foods.

Tip #34: Cultivate a mindful eating practice (and keep a food journal).

Tip #35: Relax your body to activate the vagus nerve and reduce stress-related eating.

Tip #36: Remember that where you live has powerful effects on your personal health, including body weight.

Tip #37: Observe how the social and cultural norms of the people around you influence your eating behavior.

Tip #38: Avoid or remove from your environment anything that will trigger thoughts of food.

Tip #39: Don't eat all the time. Give your body a chance to use the calories you have eaten.

Tip #40: Aim for fewer courses per meal, no snacks between or after meals, and smaller plates and portions.

Tip #41: Eat slowly. Take small bites and chew thoroughly. Don't wolf down your food.

Tip #42: Avoid the expectation effect and deprivation mindset. Don't eat food specifically labeled "diet" or "sensible" or "healthy."

Tip #43: To take your mind off food, be busy. Choose a hobby. Go outside. Call your friends.

Tip #44: Manage weight gain during celebrations and vacations by planning a week of strict eating or fasting to balance each week of holiday.

Tip #45: Eat homemade as much as possible, since you often don't know how restaurant or takeout foods are prepared.

Tip #46: To lose weight automatically, give your eating day some structure: breakfast, lunch, and dinner, no snacks.

Tip #47: Burn fat by switching between the *fed* state (eating food, high insulin) and the *fasted* state (not eating, low insulin). Fasting is the most efficient way to lower insulin.

Tip #48: Fast regularly to set up your body's expectation to burn fat, which helps make weight loss automatic.

Tip #49: Cultivate a health mindset to make healthy eating a habit.

Tip #50: Find a weight-loss buddy or join a weight-loss group.

NOTES

Preface

1   CDC. Obesity trends among U.S. adults. Behavioral Risk Factor Surveillance System (BRFSS). 1985. Available from: https://www.roswellpark.org/sites/default/files/moysich_8_29_14_obesity_trends.pdf. Accessed 2025 Sept 22.

2   Image source: Centers for Disease Control and Prevention. Percentage of American adults with BMI>30. Available from: https://www.cdc.gov/nchs/about/factsheets/factsheet_nhanes.htm. Accessed 2024 Jun 4.

Chapter 1: Debunking the Calorie Delusion

1   Mozaffarian D. Perspective: obesity—an unexplained epidemic. Am J Clin Nutr. 2022 Apr 23;115(6):1445–50. doi: 10.1093/ajcn/nqac075.

2   U.S. Department of Agriculture. Interested in losing weight? Nutrition.gov. Available from: https://www.nutrition.gov/topics/healthy-living-and-weight/strategies-success/interested-losing-weight. Accessed 2025 Aug 27.

3   Lichtenstein AH, Appel LJ, Vadiveloo M et al. 2021 Dietary guidance to improve cardiovascular health: a scientific statement from the American Heart Association. Circulation. 2021 Dec 7;144(23):e472–e487. doi: 10.1161/CIR.0000000000001031.

4   Bray GA, Bouchard C, eds. Handbook of obesity. 2nd ed. New York, Basel: Macel Dekker, Inc.; 2004. p. 126.

5   Maratos-Flier E, Flier J. Obesity. In: Kahn CR et al. Joslin's Diabetes Mellitus. 14th ed. New York: Lippincott, Williams & Wilkins; 2004. p. 541.

6   Kompaniyets L et al. Probability of 5% or greater weight loss or BMI reduction to healthy weight among adults with overweight or obesity. JAMA Netw Open. 2023;6(8):e2327358. doi: 10.1001/jamanetworkopen.2023.27358.

7   Salvia MG. The Look AHEAD trial: translating lessons learned into clinical practice and further study. Diabetes Spectr. 2017 Aug;30(3):166–70. doi: 10.2337/ds17-0016.

8   The Obesity Society. NIH stops treatment arm in the Look AHEAD trial: interpretation and implications. PR Newswire. 2012 Oct 24. Available from: https://www.prnewswire.com/news-releases/nih-stops-treatment-arm-in-the-look-ahead-trial-interpretation-and-implications-175647651.html. Accessed 2025 Oct 27.

9   Rushing J et al. Cost of intervention delivery in a lifestyle weight loss trial in type 2 diabetes: results from the Look AHEAD clinical trial. Obes Sci Pract. 2017 Feb 24;3(1):15–24. doi: 10.1002/osp4.92.

10 Wexler DJ et al. Results of a 2-year lifestyle intervention for type 2 diabetes: the Reach Ahead for Lifestyle and Health-Diabetes randomized controlled trial. Obesity (Silver Spring). 2022 Aug 31;30(10):1938–50. doi: 10.1002/oby.23508.

11 Data source for Table 1.1: DeWolfe D. Study reveals world's biggest eaters—but where does the UK rank? LBC. 2023 July 10. Available from: https://www.lbc.co.uk/article/study-reveals-worlds-biggest-eaters-but-where-does-the-uk-rank-DWz-bxQ_2/. Accessed 2025 Sept 3.

12 Ibid.

13 Image source for Figure 1.2: The obesity crisis: what does 200 calories look like?—in pictures. The Guardian. 2013 Feb 19. Available from: https://www.theguardian.com/lifeandstyle/gallery/2013/feb/19/200-calories-look-like-portion. Accessed 2025 Apr 24.

14 Speakman JR et al. Total daily energy expenditure has declined over the last 3 decades due to declining basal expenditure not reduced activity expenditure. Nat Metab. 2023 Apr 26;5(4):579–88. doi: 10.1038/s42255-023-00782-2.

15 Bays HE et al. Thirty obesity myths, misunderstandings, and/or oversimplifications: an Obesity Medicine Association (OMA) Clinical Practice Statement (CPS) 2022. Obes Pillars. 2022 Aug 10;3:100034. doi: 10.1016/j.obpill.2022.100034.

16 Pontzer H et al. Constrained total energy expenditure and metabolic adaptation to physical activity in adult humans. Curr Biol. 2016 Feb 8;26(3):410–7. doi: 10.1016/j.cub.2015.12.046.

17 Beaulieu K et al. Effect of exercise training interventions on energy intake and appetite control in adults with overweight or obesity: a systematic review and meta-analysis. Obes Rev. 2021 Jul;22 (Suppl 4):e13251. doi: 10.1111/obr.13251.

Chapter 2: Regulating the Body Fat Thermostat

1   Bray GA. The pain of weight gain: self-experimentation with overfeeding. Am J Clin Nutr. 2020 Jan 1;111(1):17–20. doi: 10.1093/ajcn/nqz264.

2   Harvard T.H. Chan School of Public Health. Healthy weight. The Nutrition Source. Available from: https://nutritionsource.hsph.harvard.edu/healthy-weight/. Accessed 2025 Mar 17.

3   Stunkard AJ. Anorectic agents lower a bodyweight set point. Life Sci. 1982;30:2043–55. doi: 10.1016/0024-3205(82)90445-3.

4   Leibel RL et al. Changes in energy expenditure resulting from altered body weight. N Engl J Med. 1995 Mar 9;332(10):621–8. doi: 10.1056/NEJM199503093321001.

5   Polidori D et al. How strongly does appetite counter weight loss? Quantification of the feedback control of human energy intake. Obesity (Silver Spring). 2016 Nov;24(11):2289–95. doi: 10.1002/oby.21653.

6   Sumithran P et al. Long-term persistence of hormonal adaptations to weight loss. N Engl J Med. 2011 Oct 27;365(17):1597–604. doi: 10.1056/NEJMoa1105816.

Chapter 3: Eating a Low-Insulin Diet

1   Hu FB et al. Trends in the incidence of coronary heart disease and changes in diet and lifestyle in women. N Engl J Med. 2000;343:530–7. doi: 10.1056/NEJM200008243430802.

2   Data source for Figure 3.1: Gross LS et al. Increased consumption of refined carbohydrates and the epidemic of type 2 diabetes in the United States: an ecologic assessment. Am J Clin Nutr. 2004 May;79(5):774–9. doi: 10.1093/ajcn/79.5.774.

3   Ibid.

4   Data source for Figure 3.5: All about the grain . . . the whole grain. Phoenix Organic Feed. Available from: https://www.phoenixorganicfeed.com/why-grind-wheat-when-i-can-buy-flour.html). Accessed 2025 Sept 3.

5   Wan Y et al. Association between changes in carbohydrate intake and long term weight changes: prospective cohort study. BMJ 2023;382:e073939. doi: 10.1136/bmj-2022-073939.

6   Ludwig DS et al. High Glycemic Index foods, overeating, and obesity. Pediatrics. 1999 Mar;103(3):E26. doi: 10.1542/peds.103.3.e26.

7   LaCombe A, Ganji V. Influence of two breakfast meals differing in glycemic load on satiety, hunger and energy intake in preschool children. Nutr J. 2010 Nov 12;9:53. doi: 10.1186/1475-2891-9-53.

8   Behall KM, Howe, JC. Effect of long-term consumption of amylose vs amylopectin starch on metabolic variables in human subjects. Am J Clin Nutr. 1995 Feb;61(2):334–40. doi: 10.1093/ajcn/61.2.334.

9   Chatterjee L, Das P. Study on amylose content of ten rice varieties recommended for Assam. Int J Pure App Biosci. 2018;6(2):1230–3. doi: 10.18782/2320-7051.6491.

10 Goddard MS et al. The effect of amylose content on insulin and glucose responses to ingested rice. Am J Clin Nutr. 1984 Mar;39(3):388–92. doi: 10.1093/ajcn/39.3.388.

11 Zhou J et al. Dietary resistant starch upregulates total GLP-1 and PYY in a sustained day-long manner through fermentation in rodents. Am J Physiol Endocrinol Metab. 2008 Nov;295(5):E1160–6. doi: 10.1152/ajpendo.90637.2008.

12 Zurbau A et al. Oat beta-glucan and postprandial blood glucose regulation: a systematic review and meta-analysis of acute, single-meal feeding, controlled trials. Curr Dev Nutr. 2020 May 29;4(Suppl 2):677. doi: 10.1093/cdn/nzaa049_070.

13 Xiong K et al. Effects of resistant starch on glycaemic control: a systematic review and meta-analysis. Br J Nutr. 2021 Jun 14;125(11):1260–9. doi: 10.1017/S0007114520003700.

14 Sonia S et al. Effect of cooling of cooked white rice on resistant starch content and glycemic response. Asia Pac J Clin Nutr. 2015;24(4):620–5. doi: 10.6133/apjcn.2015.24.4.13.

15 Chung, HY et al. Effect of partial gelatinization and retrogradation on the enzymatic digestion of waxy rice starch. J of Cereal Sci. 2006 May;43(3):353–9. doi: 10.1016/j.jcs.2005.12.001.

16 Leeman M et al. Vinegar dressing and cold storage of potatoes lowers postprandial glycaemic and insulinaemic responses in healthy subjects. Eur J Clin Nutr. 2005 Nov;59(11):1266–71. doi: 10.1038/sj.ejcn.1602238.

17 Granfeldt Y et al. On the importance of processing conditions, product thickness and egg addition for the glycaemic and hormonal responses to pasta: a comparison with bread made from "pasta ingredients." J Clin Nutr. 1991 Oct;45(10):489–99.

18 Larsen HN et al. Glycaemic index of parboiled rice depends on the severity of processing: study in type 2 diabetic subjects. Eur J Clin Nutr. 2000 May;54(5):380–5. doi: 10.1038/sj.ejcn.1600969.

19 Flood-Obbagy JE, Rolls BJ. The effect of fruit in different forms on energy intake and satiety at a meal. Appetite. 2009 April;52(2):416–22. doi: 10.1016/j.appet.2008.12.001.

20 Krishnasamy S et al. Processing apples to puree or juice speeds gastric emptying and reduces postprandial intestinal volumes and satiety in healthy adults. J Nutr. 2020 Nov 19;150(11):2890–9. doi: 10.1093/jn/nxaa191.

21 McDougall GJ et al. Different polyphenolic components of soft fruits inhibit alpha-amylase and alpha-glucosidase. Agric Food Chem. 2005 Apr 6;53(7):2760–6. doi: 10.1021/jf0489926.

22 Alkutbe R et al. Nutrient extraction lowers postprandial glucose response of fruit in adults with obesity as well as healthy weight adults. Nutrients. 2020 Mar 14;12(3):766. doi: 10.3390/nu12030766.

23 Crummett LT, Grosso RJ. Postprandial glycemic response to whole fruit versus blended fruit in healthy, young adults. Nutrients. 2022 Oct 30;14(21):4565. doi: 10.3390/nu14214565.

24 Jang C et al. The small intestine converts dietary fructose into glucose and organic acids. Cell Metab. 2018 Feb 6;27(2):351–61.e3. doi: 10.1016/j.cmet.2017.12.016.

25 Cassady BA et al. Beverage consumption, appetite, and energy intake: what did you expect? Am J Clin Nutr. 2012 Mar;95(3):587–93. doi: 10.3945/ajcn.111.025437.

26 Mattes RD, Rothacker D. Beverage viscosity is inversely related to postprandial hunger in humans. Physiol Behav. 2001 Nov–Dec;74(4–5):551–7. doi: 10.1016/s0031-9384(01)00597-2.

27 Vuksan V et al. Viscosity of fiber preloads affects food intake in adolescents. Nutr Metab Cardiovasc Dis. 2009 Sep;19(7):498–503. doi: 10.1016/j.numecd.2008.09.006.

28 Almiron-Roig E et al. Factors that determine energy compensation: a systematic review of preload studies. Nutr Rev. 2013 Jul;71(7):458–73. doi: 10.1111/nure.12048.

29 Ostman E et al. Vinegar supplementation lowers glucose and insulin responses and increases satiety after a bread meal in healthy subjects. Eur J Clin Nutr. 2005 Sep;59(9):983–8. doi: 10.1038/sj.ejcn.1602197.

30 Sugiyama M et al. Glycemic Index of single and mixed meal foods among common Japanese foods with white rice as a reference food. Eur J Clin Nutr. 2003 Jun;57(6):743–52. doi: 10.1038/sj.ejcn.1601606.

31 Freitas D et al. Glycemic response, satiety, gastric secretions and emptying after bread consumption with water, tea or lemon juice: a randomized crossover intervention using MRI. Eur J Nutr. 2022 Apr;61(3):1621–36. doi: 10.1007/s00394-021-02762-2.

32 Sugiyama M et al. Glycemic Index of single and mixed meal foods among common Japanese foods with white rice as a reference food. Eur J Clin Nutr. 2003 Jun;57(6):743–52. doi: 10.1038/sj.ejcn.1601606.

33 Collier G, O'Dea K. The effect of coingestion of fat on the glucose, insulin, and gastric inhibitory polypeptide responses to carbohydrate and protein. Am J Clin Nutr. 1983 Jun;37(6):941–4. doi: 10.1093/ajcn/37.6.941.

34 Henry CJK et al. The influence of adding fats of varying saturation on the glycaemic response of white bread. Int J Food Sci Nutr. 2008 Feb;59(1):61–9. doi: 10.1080/09637480701664183.

35 Crowe TC et al. Inhibition of enzymic digestion of amylose by free fatty acids in vitro contributes to resistant starch formation. J Nutr. 2000 Aug;130(8):2006–8. doi: 10.1093/jn/130.8.2006.

36 Owen B, Wolever T. Effect of fat on glycaemic responses in normal subjects: a dose-response study. Nutr Res. 2003 Oct;23(10):1341–7. doi: 10.1016/s0271-5317(03)00149-0.

37 Data source for Figure 3.7: Shukla AP et al. The impact of food order on postprandial glycaemic excursions in prediabetes. Diabetes Obes Metab. 2019 Feb;21(2):377–81. doi: 10.1111/dom.13503.

38 Shukla AP et al. Food order has a significant impact on postprandial glucose and insulin levels. Diabetes Care. 2015 Jun 11;38(7):e98–e99. doi: 10.2337/dc15-0429.

39 Shukla AP et al. The impact of food order on postprandial glycaemic excursions in prediabetes. Diabetes Obes Metab. 2019 Feb;21(2):377–81. doi: 10.1111/dom.13503.

40 Almoosawi S et al. Daily profiles of energy and nutrient intakes: are eating profiles changing over time? Eur J Clin Nutr. 2011 Dec 21;66(6):678–86. doi: 10.1038/ejcn.2011.210.

41 Kant AK, Graubard BI. 40-year trends in meal and snack eating behaviors of American adults. J Acad Nutr Diet. 2015 Jan;115(1):50–63. doi: 10.1016/j.jand.2014.06.354.

42 Scheer FAJ et al. The internal circadian clock increases hunger and appetite in the evening independent of food intake and other behaviors. Obesity (Silver Spring). 2013 March;21(3):421–3. doi: 10.1002/oby.20351.

43 Morgan LM et al. Effect of meal timing and glycaemic index on glucose control and insulin secretion in healthy volunteers. Br J Nutr. 2012 Oct;108(7):1286–91. doi: 10.1017/S0007114511006507.

44 Data source for Figure 3.8: Nakamura K et al. Eating dinner early improves 24-h blood glucose levels and boosts lipid metabolism after breakfast the next day: a randomized cross-over trial. Nutrients. 2021 Jul 15;13(7):2424. doi: 10.3390/nu13072424.

45 Imai S et al. Late-night-dinner deteriorates postprandial glucose and insulin whereas consuming dinner dividedly ameliorates them in patients with type 2 diabetes: a randomized crossover clinical trial. Asia Pac J Clin Nutr. 2020;29(1):68–76. doi: 10.6133/apjcn.202003_29(1).0010.

46 Madje A et al. Effects of consuming later evening meal v. earlier evening meal on weight loss during a weight loss diet: a randomised clinical trial. Br J Nutr. 2021 Aug 28;126(4):632–40. doi: 10.1017/S0007114520004456.

47 Bo S et al. Is the timing of caloric intake associated with variation in diet-induced thermogenesis and in the metabolic pattern? A randomized cross-over study. Int J Obes (Lond). 2015 Dec;39(12):1689–95. doi: 10.1038/ijo.2015.138.

48 Data source for Figure 3.9: Sutton E et al. Early time-restricted feeding improves insulin sensitivity, blood pressure, and oxidative stress even without weight loss in men with prediabetes. Cell Metab. 2018 Jun 5;27(6):1212–21.e3. doi: 10.1016/j.cmet.2018.04.010.

49 Rovira-Llopis S et al. Circadian alignment of food intake and glycaemic control by time-restricted eating: A systematic review and meta-analysis. Rev Endocr Metab Disord. 2024 Apr;25(2):325–37. doi: 10.1007/s11154-023-09853-x.

50 Jamshed H et al. Effectiveness of early time-restricted eating for weight loss, fat loss, and cardiometabolic health in adults with obesity: a randomized clinical trial. JAMA Intern Med. 2022;182(9):953–62. doi: 10.1001/jamainternmed.2022.3050.

Chapter 4: How Hormones Sustain Hunger

1   Hsu JL et al. Bariatric surgery: trends in utilization, complications, conversions and revisions. Surg Endosc. 2024 Jun 20;38(8):4613–23. doi: 10.1007/s00464-024-10985-7.

2   Dijkhorst P et al. Factors associated with decision regret after bariatric surgery. Clin Obes. 2024 Apr 14(2):e12633. doi: 10.1111/cob.12633.

3   Kelesidis T et al. Narrative review: the role of leptin in human physiology: emerging clinical applications. Ann Intern Med. 2010 Jan 19;152(2):93–100. doi: 10.7326/0003-4819-152-2-201001190-00008.

4   Shiiya T et al. Plasma ghrelin levels in lean and obese humans and the effect of glucose on ghrelin secretion. J Clin Endocrinol Metab. 2002 Jan;87(1):240–4. doi: 10.1210/jcem.87.1.8129.

5   Appleton KM et al. Sensory and physical characteristics of foods that impact food intake without affecting acceptability: systematic review and meta-analyses. Obes Rev. 2021 Aug;22(8):e13234. doi: 10.1111/obr.13234.

6   Bell EA et al. Energy density of foods affects energy intake in normal-weight women. Am J Clin Nutr. 1998 Mar;67(3):412–20. doi: 10.1093/ajcn/67.3.412.

7   Duncan KH et al. The effects of high and low energy density diets on satiety, energy intake, and eating time of obese and nonobese subjects. Am J Clin Nutr. 1983 May;37(5):763–7. doi: 10.1093/ajcn/37.5.763.

8   Ello-Martin JA et al. Dietary energy density in the treatment of obesity: a yearlong trial comparing 2 weight-loss diets. Am J Clin Nutr. 2007 Jun;85(6):1465–77. doi: 10.1093/ajcn/85.6.1465.

9   Stubbs RJ et al. The effect of covertly manipulating the energy density of mixed diets on ad libitum food intake in "pseudo free-living" humans. Int J Obes Relat Metab Disord. 1998 Oct;22(10):980–7. doi: 10.1038/sj.ijo.0800715.

10 Koren D, Taveras EM. Association of sleep disturbances with obesity, insulin resistance and the metabolic syndrome. Metabolism. 2018;84:67–75. doi: 10.1016/j.metabol.2018.04.001.

11 Lin J et al. Associations of short sleep duration with appetite-regulating hormones and adipokines: a systematic review and meta-analysis. Obes Rev. 2020 Nov;21(11):e13051. doi: 10.1111/obr.13051.

12 Schmid SM et al. A single night of sleep deprivation increases ghrelin levels and feelings of hunger in normal-weight healthy men. J Sleep Res. 2008 Sep;17(3):331–4. doi: 10.1111/j.1365-2869.2008.00662.x.

13 Van Egmond LT et al. Effects of acute sleep loss on leptin, ghrelin, and adiponectin in adults with healthy weight and obesity: a laboratory study. Obesity (Silver Spring). 2023 Mar;31(3):635–41. doi: 10.1002/oby.23616.

14 Flint A et al. Glucagon-like peptide 1 promotes satiety and suppresses energy intake in humans. J Clin Invest. 1998 Feb 1;101(3):515–20. doi: 10.1172/JCI990.

15 Nauck MA et al. Glucagon-like peptide 1 inhibition of gastric emptying outweighs its insulinotropic effects in healthy humans. Am J Physiol. 1997 Nov;273(5):E981–8. doi: 10.1152/ajpendo.1997.273.5.E981.

16 Kaufman P et al. Downsizing demand: obesity medications' impact on the food ecosystem. Morgan Stanley Research. 2023 Aug 7.

17 Flint A et al. The effect of physiological levels of glucagon-like peptide-1 on appetite, gastric emptying, energy and substrate metabolism in obesity. Int J Obes Relat Metab Disord. 2001 Jun;25(6):781–92. doi: 10.1038/sj.ijo.0801627.

18 Dockray GJ. Cholecystokinin. Curr Opin Endocrinol Diabetes Obes. 2012 Feb;19(1):8–12. doi: 10.1097/MED.0b013e32834eb77d.

19 Data source for Figure 4.3: Audrain-McGovern J, Benowitz NL. Cigarette smoking, nicotine, and body weight. Clin Pharmacol Ther. 2011 Jul;90(1):164–8. doi: 10.1038/clpt.2011.105.

20 Ibid.

21 Wadden TA et al. The fen-phen finale: a study of weight loss and valvular heart disease. Obes Res. 1998 Jul;6(4):278–84. doi: 10.1002/j.1550-8528.1998.tb00350.x.

22 Kolata G. How fen-phen, a diet "miracle," rose and fell. New York Times. 1997 Sept 23. Available from: https://www.nytimes.com/1997/09/23/science/how-fen-phen-a-diet-miracle-rose-and-fell.html. Accessed 2025 Mar 30.

23 Mayo Clinic. Beta blockers: do they cause weight gain? Mayo Clinic. 2024 April 30. https://www.mayoclinic.org/diseases-conditions/high-blood-pressure/expert-answers/beta-blockers/faq-20058385. Accessed 2025 Mar 30.

24 Gafoor R, Booth HP, Gulliford MC. Antidepressant utilisation and incidence of weight gain during 10 years' follow-up: population-based cohort study. BMJ. 2018;361(k1951):1–9. doi: 10.1136/bmj.k1951.

25 Finkelstein JS et al. Gonadal steroids and body composition, strength, and sexual function in men. N Engl J Med. 2013 Sep 12;369(11):1011–22. doi: 10.1056/NEJMoa1206168.

26 Smith MR. Changes in fat and lean body mass during androgen-deprivation therapy for prostate cancer. Urology. 2004 Apr;63(4):742–5. doi: 10.1016/j.urology.2003.10.063.

27 Wing RR et al. Weight gain at the time of menopause. Arch Intern Med. 1991 Jan;151(1):97–102.

28 Data source for Figure 4.4: Haber GB et al. Depletion and disruption of dietary fibre. Effects on satiety, plasma-glucose, and serum-insulin. Lancet. 1977 Oct 1;2(8040):679–82. doi: 10.1016/s0140-6736(77)90494-9.

29 Ibid.

30 Van der Valk ES et al. A comprehensive diagnostic approach to detect underlying causes of obesity in adults. Obes Rev. 2019 Mar 1;20(6):795–804. doi: 10.1111/obr.12836.

31 Garrow JS, Gardiner GT. Maintenance of weight loss in obese patients after jaw wiring. Br Med J (Clin Res Ed). 1981 Mar 14;282(6267):858–60. doi: 10.1136/bmj.282.6267.858.

Chapter 5: Managing Hunger, Not Calories

1 Holt SH et al. A satiety index of common foods. Eur J Clin Nutr. 1995 Sept;49:675–90.

2 Zinman B et al. Diabetes research and care through the ages. Diabetes Care 2017 Oct;40(10):1302–13. doi: 10.2337/dci17-0042.

3 Bodnaruc AM et al. Nutritional modulation of endogenous glucagon-like peptide-1 secretion: a review. Nutr Metab (Lond). 2016 Dec 9;13:92. doi: 10.1186/s12986-016-0153-3.

4 Thomsen C et al. Differential effects of saturated and monounsaturated fats on postprandial lipemia and glucagon-like peptide 1 responses in patients with type 2 diabetes. Am J Clin Nutr. 2003 Mar;77(3):605–11. doi: 10.1093/ajcn/77.3.605.

5 Paniagua JA et al. A MUFA-rich diet improves postprandial glucose, lipid and GLP-1 responses in insulin-resistant subjects. J Am Coll Nutr. 2007 Oct;26(5):434–44. doi: 10.1080/07315724.2007.10719633.

6 Essah PA et al. Effect of macronutrient composition on postprandial peptide YY levels. J Clin Endocrinol Metab. 2007 Oct;92(10):4052–5. doi: 10.1210/
   jc.2006-2273.

7 Central Committee for Medical and Community Program of the American Heart
   Association. Dietary fat and its relation to heart attacks and strokes. Report by the
   Central Committee for Medical and Community Program of the American Heart
   Association. JAMA. 1961 Feb 4;175:389–91.

8 Harcombe Z et al. Evidence from prospective cohort studies does not support
   current dietary fat guidelines: a systematic review and meta-analysis. Br J Sports
   Med. 2017 Dec;51(24):1743–9. doi: 10.1136/bjsports-2016-096550.

9 Hu FB et al. Dietary fat intake and the risk of coronary heart disease in women. N
   Engl J Med. 1997 Nov 20;337(21):1491–9. doi: 10.1056/NEJM199711203372102.

10 Dehghan M et al. Associations of fats and carbohydrate intake with cardiovascular disease and mortality in 18 countries from five continents (PURE): a
   prospective cohort study. Lancet. 2017 Nov 4;390(10107):2050–62. doi: 10.1016/
   S0140-6736(17)32252-3.

11 Poppitt SD et al. Short-term effects of macronutrient preloads on appetite and
   energy intake in lean women. Physiol Behav. 1998 Jun 1;64(3):279–85. doi:
   10.1016/s0031-9384(98)00061-4.

12 Halton TL, Hu FB. The effects of high protein diets on thermogenesis, satiety
   and weight loss: a critical review. J Am Coll Nutr. 2004 Oct;23(5):373–85. doi:
   10.1080/07315724.2004.10719381.

13 Westerterp KR et al. Diet induced thermogenesis measured over 24h in a respiration chamber: effect of diet composition. Int J Obes Relat Metab Disord. 1999
   Mar;23(3):287–92. doi: 10.1038/sj.ijo.0800810.

14 Lejeune M et al. Ghrelin and glucagon-like peptide 1 concentrations, 24-h satiety,
   and energy and substrate metabolism during a high-protein diet and measured
   in a respiration chamber. Am J Clin Nutr. 2006 Jan;83(1):89–94. doi: 10.1093/
   ajcn/83.1.89.

15 Mikkelsen PB et al. Effect of fat-reduced diets on 24-h energy expenditure: comparisons between animal protein, vegetable protein, and carbohydrate. Am J Clin
   Nutr. 2000 Nov;72(5):1135–41. doi: 10.1093/ajcn/72.5.1135.

16 Nuttall FQ, Gannon MC. Dietary protein and the blood glucose concentration. Diabetes. 2013 Apr 16;62(5):1371–2. doi: 10.2337/db12-1829.

17 Nuttall FQ et al. The metabolic response of subjects with type 2 diabetes to
   a high-protein, weight-maintenance diet. J Clin Endocrinol Metab. 2003
   Aug;88(8):3577–83. doi: 10.1210/jc.2003-030419.

18 Fromentin C et al. Dietary proteins contribute little to glucose production, even under optimal gluconeogenic conditions in healthy humans. Diabetes. 2013 Apr 16;62(5):1435–42. doi: 10.2337/db12-1208.

19 Kumar A. China tops US in daily dietary protein intake, India falls behind. Business Standard. 2024 Jul 18. Available from: https://www.business-standard.com/world-news/china-tops-us-in-daily-dietary-protein-intake-india-falls-behind-124071800427_1.html. Accessed 2025 Jan 26.

20 Kjølbæk L et al. Protein supplements after weight loss do not improve weight maintenance compared with recommended dietary protein intake despite beneficial effects on appetite sensation and energy expenditure: a randomized, controlled, double-blinded trial. Am J Clin Nutr. 2017 Aug;106(2):684–97. doi: 10.3945/ajcn.115.129528.

21 Van der Klaawu AA et al. High protein intake stimulates postprandial GLP1 and PYY release. Obesity (Silver Spring). 2013 May 13;21(8):1602–7. doi: 10.1002/oby.20154.

22 Alshamari S et al. The effect of protein supplements on weight loss, body composition, protein status, and micronutrients post laparoscopic sleeve gastrectomy (LSG): a randomised controlled trial (RCT). Ann Med Surg (Lond). 2022 Jan 1;74:103220. doi: 10.1016/j.amsu.2021.103220.

23 Kuo YY et al. Effect of whey protein supplementation in postmenopausal women: a systematic review and meta-analysis. Nutrients. 2022 Oct 10;14(19):4210. doi: 10.3390/nu14194210.

24 Rezaie P et al. Effects of bitter substances on GI function, energy intake and glycaemia—do preclinical findings translate to outcomes in humans? Nutrients. 2021 Apr 16;13(4):1317. doi: 10.3390/nu13041317.

25 Takikawa M et al. Curcumin stimulates glucagon-like peptide-1 secretion in GLU-Tag cells via Ca2+/calmodulin-dependent kinase II activation. Biochem Biophys Res Commun. 2013 May 31;435(2):165–70. doi: 10.1016/j.bbrc.2013.04.092.

26 Haldar S et al. Polyphenol-rich curry made with mixed spices and vegetables increases postprandial plasma GLP-1 concentration in a dose-dependent manner. Eur J Clin Nutr. 2018 Feb;72(2):297–300. doi: 10.1038/s41430-017-0069-7.

27 Unhapipatpong C et al. The effect of curcumin supplementation on weight loss and anthropometric indices: an umbrella review and updated meta-analyses of randomized controlled trials. Am J Clin Nutr. 2023 May;117(5):1005–16. doi: 10.1016/j.ajcnut.2023.03.006.

28 Rains TM et al. Antiobesity effects of green tea catechins: a mechanistic review. Nutr Biochem. 2011 Jan;22(1):1–7. doi: 10.1016/j.jnutbio.2010.06.006.

29 Hursel R et al. The effects of green tea on weight loss and weight mainte-
    nance: a meta-analysis. Int J Obes (Lond). 2009 Sep;33(9):956–61. doi: 10.1038/
    ijo.2009.135.

30 Rudelle S et al. Effect of a thermogenic beverage on 24-hour energy metabolism in
    humans. Obesity (Silver Spring). 2007 Feb;15(2):349–55. doi: 10.1038/oby.2007.529.

31 Dulloo AG et al. Efficacy of a green tea extract rich in catechin polyphenols and
    caffeine in increasing 24-h energy expenditure and fat oxidation in humans. Am J
    Clin Nutr. 1999 Dec;70(6):1040–5. doi: 10.1093/ajcn/70.6.1040.

32 Hursel R et al. The effects of catechin rich teas and caffeine on energy expendi-
    ture and fat oxidation: a meta-analysis. Obes Rev. 2011 Jul;12(7):e573–81. doi:
    10.1111/j.1467-789X.2011.00862.x.

33 Rumpler W et al. Oolong tea increases metabolic rate and fat oxidation in men. J
    Nutr. 2001 Nov;131(11):2848–52. doi: 10.1093/jn/131.11.2848.

34 Phung OJ et al. Effect of green tea catechins with or without caffeine on anthro-
    pometric measures: a systematic review and meta-analysis. Am J Clin Nutr. 2010
    Jan;91(1):73–81. doi: 10.3945/ajcn.2009.28157.

35 Jurgens TM et al. Green tea for weight loss and weight maintenance in overweight
    or obese adults. Cochrane Database Syst Rev. 2012 Dec 12;12(12):CD008650. doi:
    10.1002/14651858.CD008650.pub2.

36 Chen IJ et al. Therapeutic effect of high-dose green tea extract on weight reduc-
    tion: A randomized, double-blind, placebo-controlled clinical trial. Clin Nutr. 2016
    Jun;35(3):592–9. doi: 10.1016/j.clnu.2015.05.003.

37 Zhong L et al. An extract of black, green, and mulberry teas causes malabsorp-
    tion of carbohydrate but not of triacylglycerol in healthy volunteers. Am J Clin
    Nutr. 2006 Sep;84(3):551–5. doi: 10.1093/ajcn/84.3.551.

38 Bracco D et al. Effects of caffeine on energy metabolism, heart rate, and methyl-
    xanthine metabolism in lean and obese women. Am J Physiol. 1995 Oct;269(4 Pt
    1):E671–8. doi: 10.1152/ajpendo.1995.269.4.E671.

39 Henn M et al. Changes in coffee intake, added sugar and long-term weight
    gain—results from three large prospective US cohort studies. J Clin Nutr. 2023
    Dec;118(6):1164–71. doi: 10.1016/j.ajcnut.2023.09.023.

40 Van Dijk AE et al. Acute effects of decaffeinated coffee and the major coffee com-
    ponents chlorogenic acid and trigonelline on glucose tolerance. Diabetes Care.
    2009 Feb 24;32(6):1023–5. doi: 10.2337/dc09-0207.

41 Eweis DS et al. Carbon dioxide in carbonated beverages induces ghrelin release
    and increased food consumption in male rats: implications on the onset of obesity.
    Obes Res Clin Pract. 2017 Sep-Oct;11(5):534–43. doi: 10.1016/j.orcp.2017.02.001.

42 Colditz GA et al. Patterns of weight change and their relation to diet in a cohort of healthy women. Am J Clin Nutr. 1990 Jun;51(6):1100–5. doi: 10.1093/ajcn/51.6.1100.

43 Fowler SP et al. Fueling the obesity epidemic? Artificially sweetened beverage use and long-term weight gain. Obesity (Silver Spring). 2008 Aug;16(8):1894–900. doi: 10.1038/oby.2008.284.

44 Azad MB et al. Nonnutritive sweeteners and cardiometabolic health: a systematic review and meta-analysis of randomized controlled trials and prospective cohort studies. CMAJ. 2017 Jul 17;189(28):E929–39. doi: 10.1503/cmaj.161390.

45 Eweis DS et al. Carbon dioxide in carbonated beverages induces ghrelin release and increased food consumption in male rats: implications on the onset of obesity. Obes Res Clin Pract. 2017 Sep-Oct;11(5):534–43. doi: 10.1016/j.orcp.2017.02.001.

46 Chakravartti SP et al. Non-caloric sweetener effects on brain appetite regulation in individuals across varying body weights. Nat Metab. 2025;7:574–85. doi: 10.1038/s42255-025-01227-8.

47 WHO. WHO advises not to use non-sugar sweeteners for weight control in newly released guideline. News, World Health Organization. 2023 May 15. Available from: https://www.who.int/news/item/15-05-2023-who-advises-not-to-use-non-sugar-sweeteners-for-weight-control-in-newly-released-guideline. Accessed 2025 Mar 30.

48 Holt SH et al. The effects of sugar-free vs sugar-rich beverages on feelings of fullness and subsequent food intake. Int J Food Sci Nutr. 2000 Jan;51(1):59–71. doi: 10.1080/096374800100912.

49 Holt SH et al. The effects of equal-energy portions of different breads on blood glucose levels, feelings of fullness and subsequent food intake. J Am Diet Assoc. 2001 Jul;101(7):767–73. doi: 10.1016/S0002-8223(01)00192-4.

50 Fazzino TL et al. Ad libitum meal energy intake is positively influenced by energy density, eating rate and hyper-palatable food across four dietary patterns. Nat Food. 2023 Feb;4(2):144–7. doi: 10.1038/s43016-022-00688-4.

Chapter 6: Getting Hooked On Ultra-Processed Foods

1 Dietary guidelines: the Food Guide Pyramid is demolished. World Public Health Nutrition Association. 2011 June. Available from: https://www.wphna.org/htdocs/2011_june_hp0_food_pyramid.htm. Accessed 2025 Aug 27.

2 Gutierrez-Ortiz C et al. Impact of ultra-processed foods consumption on the burden of obesity and type 2 diabetes in Belgium: a comparative risk assessment. BMC Public Health. 2025 Mar 22;25(1):1097. doi: 10.1186/s12889-025-22304-3.

3   Juul F et al. Ultra-processed food consumption among US adults from 2001 to 2018. Am J Clin Nutr. 2022 Jan 11;115(1):211–21. doi: 10.1093/ajcn/nqab305.

4   Data source for Figure 6.1: Stearn E. Proof not ALL ultraprocessed foods are bad for you? Ready meals, vegan substitutes and cereals DON'T cause cancer or diabetes, huge study claims. Daily Mail. 2023 Nov 13. Available from: https://www.dailymail.co.uk/health/article-12744029/Proof-not-ultraprocessed-foods-bad-Ready-meals-vegan-substitutes-cereals-DONT-cause-cancer-diabetes-huge-study-claims.html. Accessed 2025 Aug 27.

5   Ibid.

6   Hall KH et al. Ultra-processed diets cause excess calorie intake and weight gain: an inpatient randomized controlled trial of ad libitum food intake. Cell Metab. 2019 Jul 2;30(1):67–77.e3. doi: 10.1016/j.cmet.2019.05.008.

7   Lee JH et al. United States dietary trends since 1800: lack of association between saturated fatty acid consumption and non-communicable diseases. Front Nutr. 2022 Jan 13;8:748847. doi: 10.3389/fnut.2021.748847.

8   Beggs A. Diet foods of the '80s are out. But has anything really changed? Bon Appétit. 2022 Jan 10. Available from: https://www.bonappetit.com/story/diet-food-in-america. Accessed 2025 Aug 27.

9   Data source for Figure 6.3: Wood et al. What is the purpose of ultra-processed food? An exploratory analysis of the financialisation of ultra-processed food corporations and implications for public health. Global Health. 2023 Nov 13;19(1):85. doi: 10.1186/s12992-023-00990-1.

10   Ibid.

11   Gompertz S. How did households budget in 1957? BBC. 2018 Jan 18. Available from: https://www.bbc.com/news/business-42735294. Accessed 2025 Aug 27.

12   Sweitzer M, Davidenko V. Food accounted for 12.9 percent of U.S. households' expenditures in 2023. Available from: https://www.ers.usda.gov/data-products/chart-gallery/chart-detail?chartId=58276. Accessed 2025 Aug 27.

13   Ravandi B et al. Prevalence of processed foods in major U.S. grocery stores. Nat Food. 2025 Mar;6(3):296–308. doi: 10.1038/s43016-024-01095-7.

14   Zhong A et al. The marketing of ultraprocessed foods in a national sample of U.S. supermarket circulars: a pilot study. AJPM Focus. 2022 Jun 29;1(1):100009. doi: 10.1016/j.focus.2022.100009.

15   Chen ZH et al. Ultraprocessed food consumption and obesity development in Canadian children. JAMA Netw Open. 2025 Jan 2;8(1):e2457341. doi: 10.1001/jamanetworkopen.2024.57341.

16 Ministry of Health of Brazil, Secretariat of Health Care, Primary Health Care Department. Dietary guidelines for the Brazilian population. Brasilia: Ministry of Health of Brazil; 2015. Available from: https://bvsms.saude.gov.br/bvs/publicacoes/dietary_guidelines_brazilian_population.pdf. Accessed 2025 Aug 27.

17 Pollan M. Food rules: an eater's manual. New York: Penguin; 2009.

18 Marino M et al. A systematic review of worldwide consumption of ultra-processed foods: findings and criticisms. Nutrients. 2021 Aug 13;13(8):2778. doi: 10.3390/nu13082778.

19 CDC Public Health. Adult obesity facts. CDC. 2024 May 14. Available from: https://www.cdc.gov/obesity/adult-obesity-facts/index.html. Accessed 2025 Aug 27.

20 Percentage of obese individuals in Italy in 2023, by gender and age. Statista. Available from: https://www.statista.com/statistics/1319198/share-of-obese-individuals-in-italy-by-gender-and-age/. Accessed 2025 Aug 27.

21 What is ultra-processed food and what does it mean for my health? BBC Food. 2025 April. Available from: https://www.bbc.co.uk/food/articles/what_is_ultra-processed_food. Accessed 2025 Aug 27.

22 Rauber F et al. Ultra-processed food consumption and chronic non-communicable diseases-related dietary nutrient profile in the UK (2008–2014). Nutrients. 2018 May 9;10(5):587. doi: 10.3390/nu10050587.

23 Ravandi B et al. Prevalence of processed foods in major US grocery stores. Nat Food. 2025 Jan 13. doi: 10.1038/s43016-024-01095-7.

Chapter 7: Understanding Food Addiction

1 The price of smoking for a lifetime is lowest in the South, highest in the Northeast: here are the numbers. The Cancer Letter. 2020 Jan 24;46(4). Available from: https://cancerletter.com/the-cancer-letter/20200124_4. Accessed 2025 Aug 27.

2 Wheelwright T. Cell phone usage stats 2025: Americans check their phones 205 times a day. Reviews.org. 2025 Jan 1. Available from: https://www.reviews.org/mobile/cell-phone-addiction/. Accessed 2025 Aug 27.

3 Fitzgerald K. Why alcohol is the deadliest drug. Addiction Center. Available from: https://www.addictioncenter.com/community/why-alcohol-is-the-deadliest-drug/. Accessed 2025 Aug 27.

4 Mazerolle J. The long struggle for cigarette warnings has lessons for alcohol labels, experts say. CBC News. 2023 Jan 19. Available from: https://www.cbc.ca/news/canada/cigarette-warning-labels-cancer-alcohol-1.6716405. Accessed 2025 Aug 27.

5 DiFranza JR et al. RJR Nabisco's cartoon camel promotes Camel cigarettes to children. JAMA. 1991 Dec 11;266(22):3149–53.

6   Fischer PM et al. Brand logo recognition by children aged 3 to 6 years: Mickey Mouse and Old Joe the Camel. JAMA. 1991 Dec 11;266(22):3145–8.

7   UConn Rudd Center for Food Policy and Health. Food marketing. Available from: https://uconnruddcenter.org/research/food-marketing/. Accessed 2025 Aug 27.

8   Philip Morris. Proposal for the organisation of the Whitecoat Project. 25 June 2002. Truth Tobacco Industry Documents, Bates no. 3990006961-3990006964. Available from: https://www.industrydocuments.ucsf.edu/tobacco/docs/#id=kynp0183. Accessed 2025 Aug 27.

9   Kearns CE et al. Sugar industry and coronary heart disease research: a historical analysis of internal industry documents. JAMA Intern Med. 2016 Nov 1;176(11):1680–5. doi: 10.1001/jamainternmed.2016.5394.

10 Schillinger D et al. Do sugar-sweetened beverages cause obesity and diabetes? Industry and the manufacture of scientific controversy. Ann Intern Med. 2016 Dec 20;165(12):895–7. doi: 10.7326/L16-0534.

11 Blackwell T. Canadian researchers have received hundreds of thousands from soft-drink makers and the sugar industry. National Post. 2015 Dec 6. Available from: https://nationalpost.com/health/canadian-researchers-have-received-hundreds-of-thousands-from-soft-drink-makers-and-the-sugar-industry. Accessed 2025 Aug 27.

12 O'Connor A. University returns $1 million grant to Coca-Cola. The New York Times. 2015 Nov 6. Available from: https://archive.nytimes.com/well.blogs.nytimes.com/2015/11/06/university-returns-1-million-grant-to-coca-cola/. Accessed 2025 Aug 27.

13 Steele EM et al. Ultra-processed foods and added sugars in the US diet: evidence from a nationally representative cross-sectional study. BMJ Open. 2016 Jan 4;6(3):e009892. doi: 10.1136/bmjopen-2015-009892.

14 Schulte EM et al. Which foods may be addictive? The roles of processing, fat content, and glycemic load. PLoS One. 2015 Feb 18;10(2):e0117959. doi: 10.1371/journal.pone.0117959.

15 Gearhardt A et al. Social, clinical, and policy implications of ultra-processed food addiction BMJ. 2023;383:e075354. doi: 10.1136/bmj-2023-075354.

16 Data source for Figure 7.1: Brewerton TD. Food addiction as a proxy for eating disorder and obesity severity, trauma history, PTSD symptoms, and comorbidity. Eat Weight Disord. 2017 Jun;22(2):241–7. doi: 10.1007/s40519-016-0355-8.

17 Ibid.

18 Pursey KM et al. The prevalence of food addiction as assessed by the Yale Food Addiction Scale: a systematic review. Nutrients. 2014 Oct 21;6(10):4552–90. doi: 10.3390/nu6104552.

19 Camacho-Barcia L et al. Metabolic, affective and neurocognitive characterization of metabolic syndrome patients with and without food addiction: implications for weight progression. Nutrients. 2021 Aug 13;13(8):2779. doi: 10.3390/nu13082779.

20 Silva Júnior AE, Macena ML, Bueno NB. The prevalence of food addiction and its association with type 2 diabetes: a systematic review with meta-analysis. Br J Nutr. 2025 Feb 28;133(4):558–66. doi:10.1017/S000711452500008X.

21 Burmeister JM et al. Food addiction in adults seeking weight loss treatment: implications for psychosocial health and weight loss. Appetite. 2013 Jan;60(1):103–10. doi: 10.1016/j.appet.2012.09.013.

22 Gearhardt AN et al. The neural correlates of "food addiction." Arch Gen Psychiatry. 2011 Apr 4;68(8):808–16. doi: 10.1001/archgenpsychiatry.2011.32.

23 Randolph TG. The descriptive features of food addiction; addictive eating and drinking. Q J Stud Alcohol. 1956 Jun;17(2):198–224. doi: 10.15288/qjsa.1956.17.198.

24 DiFeliceantonio AG et al. Supra-additive effects of combining fat and carbohydrate on food reward. Cell Metab. 2018 Jul 3;28(1):33–44.e3. doi: 10.1016/j.cmet.2018.05.018.

25 Schulte EM et al. Which foods may be addictive? The roles of processing, fat content, and glycemic load. PLoS One. 2015 Feb 18;10(2):e0117959. doi: 10.1371/journal.pone.0117959.

26 Lennerz B, Lennerz JK. Food addiction, high-Glycemic-Index carbohydrates, and obesity. Clin Chem. 2018 Jan;64(1):64–71. doi: 10.1373/clinchem.2017.273532.

27 Martin CK et al. Changes in food cravings during low-calorie and very-low-calorie diets. Obesity (Silver Spring). 2006 Jan;14(1):115–21. doi: 10.1038/oby.2006.14.

28 Lappalainen R et al. Hunger/craving responses and reactivity to food stimuli during fasting and dieting. Int J Obes. 1990 Aug;14(8):679–88.

29 Kahathuduwa CN et al. Extended calorie restriction suppresses overall and specific food cravings: a systematic review and a meta-analysis. Obes Rev. 2017 Oct;18(10):1122-1135. doi: 10.1111/obr.12566.

30 Unwin J et al. Low carbohydrate and psychoeducational programs show promise for the treatment of ultra-processed food addiction: 12-month follow-up. Front Psychiatry. Sec. Addictive Disorders;2025 13 April;16. doi: 10.3389/fpsyt.2025.1556988.

Chapter 8: Managing Emotional Eating

1   Gay R. Hunger: a memoir of (my) body. New York: Harper; 2017.

2   Fasano A. The physiology of hunger. N Engl J Med 2025;392(4):372–81. doi: 10.1056/NEJMra2402679.

3   Wong L et al. Emotional eating in patients attending a specialist obesity treatment service. Appetite. 2020;151:104708. doi: 10.1016/j.appet.2020.104708.

4   Van Strien T, Oosterveld P. The children's DEBQ for assessment of restrained, emotional and external eating in 7- to 12-year-old children. Int J Eat Disord. 2008 Jan;41:72–81. doi: 10.1002/eat.20424.

5   Van Strien T. Causes of emotional eating and matched treatment of obesity. Curr Diab Rep. 2018 Apr 25;18(6):35. doi: 10.1007/s11892-018-1000-x.

6   Stouffer MA et al. Insulin enhances striatal dopamine release by activating cholinergic interneurons and thereby signals reward. Nat Commun. 2015 Oct 27;6:8543. doi: 10.1038/ncomms9543.

7   Ozier AD et al. Overweight and obesity are associated with emotion- and stress-related eating as measured by the Eating and Appraisal Due to Emotions and Stress Questionnaire. J Am Diet Assoc. 2008 Jan;108(1):49–56. doi: 10.1016/j.jada.2007.10.011.

8   Anglé S et al. Three factor eating questionnaire-R18 as a measure of cognitive restraint, uncontrolled eating and emotional eating in a sample of young Finnish females. Int J Behav Nutr Phys Act. 2009 Jul 17;6:41. doi: 10.1186/1479-5868-6-41.

9   Rahme C et al. Emotional eating among Lebanese adults: scale validation, prevalence and correlates. Eat Weight Disord. 2021 May;26(4):1069–78.

10 Raman J et al. The clinical obesity maintenance model: an integration of psychological constructs including mood, emotional regulation, disordered overeating, habitual cluster behaviours, health literacy and cognitive function. J Obes. 2013 Feb 14;2013:240128. doi: 10.1155/2013/240128.

11 Renn BN et al. The bidirectional relationship of depression and diabetes: a systematic review. Clin Psychol Rev. 2011 Dec;31(8):1239–46. doi: 10.1016/j.cpr.2011.08.001.

12 Tumin R, Anderson SE. Television, home-cooked meals, and family meal frequency: associations with adult obesity. J Acad Nutr Diet. 2017 Jun;117(6):937–45.

13 Robinson E et al. Eating attentively: a systematic review and meta-analysis of the effect of food intake memory and awareness on eating. Am J Clin Nutr. 2013 Apr;97(4):728–42. doi: 10.3945/ajcn.112.045245.

14 Duif I et al. Effects of distraction on taste-related neural processing: a cross-sectional fMRI study. Am J Clin Nutr. 2020;111(5):950–61. doi: 10.1093/ajcn/nqaa032.

15 Rozin P et al. What causes humans to begin and end a meal? A role for memory for what has been eaten, as evidenced by a study of multiple meal eating in amnesic patients. Psychol Sci. 1998;9(5):392–396. doi: 10.1111/1467-9280.00073.

16 Rogers JM et al. Mindfulness-based interventions for adults who are overweight or obese: a meta-analysis of physical and psychological health outcomes. Obes Rev. 2017 Jan;18(1):51–67. doi: 10.1111/obr.12461.

17 Carrière K et al. Mindfulness-based interventions for weight loss: a systematic review and meta-analysis. Obes Rev. 2018 Feb;19(2):164–77. doi: 10.1111/obr.12623.

18 Paturel A. Bolster your brain by stimulating the vagus nerve. Cedars Sinai Blog. 2024 Mar 21. Available from: https://www.cedars-sinai.org/blog/stimulating-the-vagus-nerve.html. Accessed 2025 Apr 7.

19 Chevalier G et al. Earthing: Health implications of reconnecting the human body to the Earth's surface electrons. J Environ Public Health. 2012 Jan 12;2012:291541. doi: 10.1155/2012/291541.

20 Cluskey M, Grobe D. College weight gain and behavior transitions: male and female differences. J Am Diet Assoc. 2009 Feb;109:325–9. doi: 10.1016/j.jada.2008.10.045.

21 Sobal J et al. Gender, ethnicity, marital status, and body weight in the United States. Obesity (Silver Spring). 2009 Dec;17(12):2223–31. doi: 10.1038/oby.2009.64.

22 Leeners et al. Ovarian hormones and obesity. Hum Reprod Update. 2017 May 1;23(3):300–21. doi: 10.1093/humupd/dmw045.

Chapter 9: Living in an Obesogenic Environment

1 Ng, M et al. National-level and state-level prevalence of overweight and obesity among children, adolescents, and adults in the USA, 1990–2021, and forecasts up to 2050. Lancet. 2024 Dec 7;404(10469):2278–98. doi: 10.1016/S0140-6736(24)01548-4.

2 DeWolfe D. Study reveals world's biggest eaters—but where does the UK rank? LBC. 2023 July 10. Available from:https://www.lbc.co.uk/news/study-reveals-worlds-biggest-eaters-but-where-does-the-uk-rank/. Accessed 2025 Aug 27.

3 Goel MS et al. Obesity among US immigrant subgroups by duration of residence. JAMA. 2004 Dec 15;292(23):2860–7. doi: 10.1001/jama.292.23.2860.

4   Yoneda M et al. A 50-year history of the health impacts of Westernization on the lifestyle of Japanese Americans: a focus on the Hawaii–Los Angeles–Hiroshima Study. J Diabetes Investig. 2020 May 26;11(6):1382–7. doi: 10.1111/jdi.13278.

5   Curb JD, Markus EB. Body fat and obesity in Japanese Americans. Am J Clin Nutr. 1991 Jun;53(6 Suppl):1552S–5S. doi: 10.1093/ajcn/53.6.1552S.

6   Shikany JM et al. Southern dietary pattern is associated with hazard of acute coronary heart disease in the Reasons for Geographic and Racial Differences in Stroke (REGARDS) study. Circulation. 2015 Sep 1;132(9):804–14. doi: 10.1161/ CIRCULATIONAHA.114.014421.

7   Percentage of adults with obesity in the United States as of 2023, by state. Statista. Available from: https://www.statista.com/statistics/378988/us-obesity-rate-by-state/. Accessed 2025 Aug 27.

8   Malinsky G. 57% of Gen Zers want to be influencers—but "it's constant, Monday through Sunday," says creator. CNBC Make It. 2024 Sep 14. Available from: https:// www.cnbc.com/2024/09/14/more-than-half-of-gen-z-want-to-be-influencers-but-its-constant.html. Accessed 2025 Apr 25.

9   Datar A et al. Association of exposure to communities with high obesity with body type norms and obesity risk among teenagers. JAMA Netw Open. 2020 Mar 2;3(3):e200846. doi: 10.1001/jamanetworkopen.2020.0846.

10 Christakis NA, Fowler JH. The spread of obesity in a large social network over 32 years. N Engl J Med. 2007 Jul 26;357(4):370–9. doi: 10.1056/NEJMsa066082.

11 Popkin BM et al. Does hunger and satiety drive eating anymore? Increasing eating occasions and decreasing time between eating occasions in the United States. Am J Clin Nutr. 2010 May;91(5):1342–7. doi: 10.3945/ajcn.2009.28962.

12 Data source for Figure 9.1: What is ultra-processed food and what does it mean for my health? BBC Food. 2019 June. Available from: https://www.bbc.co.uk/food/ articles/what_is_ultra-processed_food. Accessed 2025 Oct 22.

13 Smeets P et al. Cephalic phase responses and appetite. Nutr Rev. 2010 Nov;68(11):643–55. doi: 10.1111/j.1753-4887.2010.00334.x.

14 Data source for Figure 9.2: USAFacts team. Federal farm subsidies: what the data says. USAFacts. Available from: https://usafacts.org/articles/federal-farm-subsidies-what-data-says/. Accessed 2025 Jul 18.

15 Ibid.

16 Siegel KR et al. Association of higher consumption of foods derived from subsidized commodities with adverse cardiometabolic risk among US adults. JAMA Intern Med. 2016 Aug 1;176(8):1124–32. doi: 10.1001/jamainternmed.2016.2410.

17 Piñeiro V, Soto D. Policy seminar: the harmful environment impacts of agricultural subsidies and prospects for reform. IFPRI Blog. 2023 Jan 6. Available from: https://www.ifpri.org/blog/policy-seminar-harmful-environment-impacts-agricultural-subsidies-and-prospects-reform/. Accessed 2025 Aug 27.

18 Fletcher ER. World sees "unprecedented" hunger as farm subsidies boost unhealthy foods. Health Policy Watch. 2022 June 7. Available from: https://healthpolicy-watch.news/world-sees-unprecedented-hunger-as-farm-subsidies-boost-unhealthy-foods/. Accessed 2025 Aug 27.

19 Wolf K. 35 key food & beverage marketing statistics. Champ Digital blog. Undated. Available from: https://champdigital.com/blog/food-beverage-marketing-statistics/. Accessed 2025 Aug 27.

Chapter 10: Recognizing Eating as a Habit

1 Apolzan JW et al. Frequency of consuming foods predicts changes in cravings for those foods during weight loss: the POUNDS Lost study. Obesity (Silver Spring). 2017 Jun 15;25(8):1343–8. doi: 10.1002/oby.21895.

2 Data source for Figure 10.1: Natalucci G et al. Spontaneous 24-h ghrelin secretion pattern in fasting subjects: maintenance of a meal-related pattern. Eur J Endocrinol. 2005 Jun;152(6):845–50. doi: 10.1530/eje.1.01919.

3 Ibid.

4 Kant AK, Graubard BI. 40-year trends in meal and snack eating behaviors of American adults. J Acad Nutr Diet. 2015 Jan;115(1):50–63. doi: 10.1016/j.jand.2014.06.354.

5 Dietary Guidelines Advisory Committee. Scientific report of the 2020 Dietary Guidelines Advisory Committee: advisory report to the Secretary of Agriculture and the Secretary of Health and Human Services. Washington, DC: U.S. Department of Agriculture, Agricultural Research Service; 2020 July. pp. 13, 719. Available from: https://www.dietaryguidelines.gov/sites/default/files/2020-07/Scientific Report_of_the_2020DietaryGuidelinesAdvisoryCommittee_first-print.pdf. Accessed 2025 Aug 27.

6 Natalucci G et al. Spontaneous 24-h ghrelin secretion pattern in fasting subjects: maintenance of a meal-related pattern. Eur J Endocrinol. 2005 Jun;152(6):845–50. doi: 10.1530/eje.1.01919.

7 Espelund U et al. Fasting unmasks a strong inverse association between ghrelin and cortisol in serum: studies in obese and normal-weight subjects. J Clin Endocrinol Metab. 2005 Feb 1;90(2): 741–46. doi: 10.1210/jc.2004-0604.

8 Young LR, Nestle M. The contribution of expanding portion sizes to the US obesity epidemic. Am J Public Health. 2002 Feb;92(2):246–9. doi: 10.2105/ajph.92.2.246.

9   Large portion sizes contribute to U.S. obesity problem. National Heart, Lung, and Blood Institute. We Can! Community News Feature. Available from: https://www.nhlbi.nih.gov/health/educational/wecan/news-events/matte1.htm. Accessed 2025 Jan 1.

10   Ruby MB et al. Differences in portion sizes in Brazil, France, and the USA. Foods. 2024 Feb 1;13(3):455. doi: 10.3390/foods13030455.

11   Hawton K et al. Slow down: behavioural and physiological effects of reducing eating rate. Nutrients. 2018 Dec 27;11(1):50. doi: 10.3390/nu11010050.

12   Karl JP et al. Independent and combined effects of eating rate and energy density on energy intake, appetite, and gut hormones. Obesity (Silver Spring). 2013;21:E244–52. doi: 10.1002/oby.20075.

13   Shah M et al. Slower eating speed lowers energy intake in normal-weight but not overweight/obese subjects. J Acad Nutr Diet. 2014 Mar;114(3):393–402. doi: 10.1016/j.jand.2013.11.002.

14   Jonas WB et al. To what extent are surgery and invasive procedures effective beyond a placebo response? A systematic review with meta-analysis of randomised, sham controlled trials. BMJ Open. 2015 Dec 11;5(12):e009655. doi: 10.1136/bmjopen-2015-009655.

15   Crum AJ et al. Mind over milkshakes: mindsets, not just nutrients, determine ghrelin response. Health Psychol. 2011 Jul;30(4):424–9; discussion 430–1. doi: 10.1037/a0023467.

16   Arosio, M et al. Effects of modified sham feeding on ghrelin levels in healthy human subjects. J Clin Endocrinol Metab. 2004 Oct;89(10):5101–4. doi: 10.1210/jc.2003-032222.

17   Finkelstein SR, Fishbach A. When healthy food makes you hungry. J Consum Res. 2010 Oct;37(3):357–67. doi: 10.1086/652248.

18   Turnwald BP et al. Increasing vegetable intake by emphasizing tasty and enjoyable attributes: a randomized controlled multisite intervention for taste-focused labeling. Psychol Sci. 2019 Nov;30(11):1603–15. doi: 10.1177/0956797619872191.

19   Watson S et al. The power of suggestion: subjective satiety is affected by nutrient and health-focused food labelling with no effect on physiological gut hormone release. Nutrients. 2022 Dec 1;14(23):5100. doi: 10.3390/nu14235100.

20   Brown SD et al. We are what we (think we) eat: The effect of expected satiety on subsequent calorie consumption. Appetite. 2020 Sept 1;152:104717. doi: 10.1016/j.appet.2020.104717.

21   Helander EE et al. Weight gain over the holidays in three countries. N Engl J Med. 2016;375:1200–2. doi: 10.1056/NEJMc1602012.

22 Cooper JA, Tokar T. A prospective study on vacation weight gain in adults. Physiol Behav. 2016 Mar 15;156:43–7. doi: 10.1016/j.physbeh.2015.12.028.

23 Houben K, Dibbets P. Taming temptations: comparing the effectiveness of counterconditioning and extinction in reducing food cue reactivity. Appetite. 2025 Apr 1;208:107932. doi: 10.1016/j.appet.2025.107932.

Chapter 11: Making Weight Loss Automatic

1 Wang Z et al. Trends in Chinese snacking behaviors and patterns and the social-demographic role between 1991 and 2009. Asia Pac J Clin Nutr. 2012;21(2):253–62.

2 Gill S, Panda S. A smartphone app reveals erratic diurnal eating patterns in humans that can be modulated for health benefits. Cell Metab. 2015 Nov 3;22(5):789–98. doi: 10.1016/j.cmet.2015.09.005.

3 Jamshed H et al. Effectiveness of early time-restricted eating for weight loss, fat loss, and cardiometabolic health in adults with obesity. JAMA Intern Med. 2022 Aug 8;182(9):953–62. doi: 10.1001/jamainternmed.2022.3050.

4 Kahleova H et al. Meal frequency and timing are associated with changes in Body Mass Index in Adventist Health Study 2. J Nutr. 2017 Sep;147(9):1722–8. doi: 10.3945/jn.116.244749.

Chapter 12: Unlocking the Secrets of Success—Your Mindset and Your Habits

1 Keeping a step ahead: men in Osaka and women in Kanagawa score top for walking. Nippon.com. 2019 Jan 22. Available from: https://www.nippon.com/en/japan-data/h00372/keeping-a-step-ahead-men-in-osaka-and-women-in-kanagawa-score-top-for-walking.html. Accessed 2025 Aug 8.

2 Dailey R et al. The buddy benefit: increasing the effectiveness of an employee-targeted weight-loss program. J Health Commun. 2018;23(3):272–80. doi: 10.1080/10810730.2018.1436622.

Chapter 13: Putting the Golden Rules of Weight Loss Into Action

1 Winfrey O. My 67-pound weight loss (1988). Oprah.com, Oprah's top 20 moments. Available from: https://www.oprah.com/oprahshow/oprahs-top-20-moments. Accessed 2025 Apr 14.

2 Clear J. Atomic habits: an easy & proven way to build good habits & break bad ones. New York: Avery; 2018.

INDEX

exercise, 18–20, 74, 146, 201–2
expectation effect, 174–76
eyes, 27

fasting: benefits, 222; daily, 191–93;
early time-restricted eating, 61;
The Fasting Method online community, 213; fed state vs. fasted
state, 193–95; food addiction
and, 133; frequency and length,
229; ghrelin and, 170–71;
Gloria's experience, 149; Golden
Rule (regularity), 197–98, 222;
hypoglycemia and, 77–78; insulin and, 14; Lindy Effect and,
224; reframing, 204–5; skipping
a meal, 195–97
fat oxidation, 88, 89. *See also* body
fat; body fat thermostat; dietary
fat; lipolysis
fatty liver, 55
feelings, 200. *See also* mindset
fenfluramine, 33, 73
fen-phen, 73, 79
fermented foods, 56, 226
fiber, 43, 48–50, 54, 68, 105
fish, 37, 83, 92, 225. *See also* seafood
flavors, artificial, 93, 112, 118, 123
Flier, Jeffrey, 5
food: about, 42; acidic and fermented, 56, 226; avoiding foods
with labels, 120; bitter, 86–87;
bulky, 67–68; comfort, 138; cues
and triggers, 161–63; energy-
dense, 93; fattening, 14, 35; food
preparation, 53–55; food processing, 43–44; food viscosity,
55–56; heavy, 68; hormones
and, xvi–xvii, 9–11, 35–36;
hyper-palatable, 93; Lindy Effect

and, 223–24; "low fat" or "fat
free," 83–84; low-insulin diet,
62–63, 225–26; misguided
dietary advice, 37–38, 82, 109–
11; NOVA classification system,
100–102; "nutrient-dense," 68;
plant-based, 85, 227; protein
powders, 85–86; satiety and,
80–81. *See also* absorption;
carbohydrates; dietary fat;
digestion; drinks; eating; protein; ultra-processed foods
food addiction: characteristics
of addictive foods, 130–32;
comparison to food cravings,
132–33; prevalence, 129–30;
signs of, 132; treatment, 133–34;
ultra-processed foods, 120, 123–
26. *See also* addiction
food dyes, artificial, 119
food matrix, 51–52, 86, 106, 124
forest bathing, 146
France, 82, 172
french fries, 68, 113–14
fructose, 55. *See also* high-fructose
corn syrup
fruit, 54–55, 226

gastric (stomach) emptying, 53, 54,
55, 57, 67–68, 70, 71
Gay, Roxane, 135, 136
gender. *See* men; women
General Foods, 126
genetically modified foods, 119
Germany, 8, 39, 177
ghrelin: about, 13, 34, 66–67; bitter
foods and, 86; as conditioned
response, 168; eating slowly and,
173; expectation effect, 162, 175;
fasting and, 170–71, 197; green

life changes, 147–48
lifestyles, active, 211
Lindy Effect, 223–24
lipolysis, 14, 16, 72, 194. *See also* body fat
liver, fatty, 55
low-calorie sweeteners (LCS), 90–91. *See also* artificial sweeteners

maltodextrin, 123
mango, 54–55
Maratos-Flier, Eleftheria, 5
marketing, 115, 127, 134, 164, 221
marriage, 147
massage, 147
McDonald's, 113–14
meals. *See* eating
meat, 103, 225. *See also* protein
meditation, 146
megestrol, 33, 75
melanin-concentrating hormone, 67
men, 33, 69, 73, 74–75, 147
menopause, 75, 148
menstrual cycle, 75, 147–48
metabolic rate, 15, 18–19, 28, 30–31, 60, 76, 88
metabolism, 41–42, 61, 84, 87, 88, 89. *See also* absorption; digestion
methamphetamine (speed), 73, 79. *See also* amphetamines
Mexico, 160
mindful eating, 142–45, 211–12, 229. *See also* emotional eating
mindless (distracted) eating, 140–41, 160
mindset: Golden Rule (commitment), 214, 222; importance of, 199–200; management and developing, 200–202; reframing fasting and snacking, 204–5;

reframing ultra-processed foods, 203–4
modified starches, 119
monosodium glutamate (MSG), 123
Monteiro, Carlos, 99–100
Mounjaro (tirzepatide), 71, 79
Mozaffarian, Dariush, 3, 7
mushrooms, 49, 226, 227
My 600-lb Life (TV show), 64

Nabisco, 126
National Health and Nutrition Examination Survey, 191
nature walking, 146
Nestle, Marion, 128
Neumann, Rudolf, 24
neurotransmitter spike, 124–25
New Zealand, 119
nicotine, 33, 72, 79, 121, 124, 125. *See also* smoking
noradrenaline, 33, 72, 88, 197
norepinephrine, 13, 73
NOVA food classification system, 100–102
Nurses' Health Study, 91
nut milks, 227
"nutrient-dense" foods, 68
nuts and seeds, 37, 57, 225

oat bran, 50
oat milk, 227
oats (oatmeal), 45–46, 48, 49
obesity. *See* weight gain
The Obesity Code (Fung), xiii, 5, 32, 55, 81, 193, 221, 222, 230
oils: olive, 56, 81; seed, 82–83, 119
olives, 55
orexin, 67
Osler, William, 81
overfeeding studies, 24–25, 34

social modeling (social cues),
158–60, 177, 220, 225. *See also*
conditioned hunger; habits
sodas, diet, 90–91, 132
soups, 55–56, 112, 118, 228
sourdough, 46
South Africa, 160
South Korea, 160
soy milk, 227
sparkling water, 90
speed (methamphetamine), 73, 79.
See also amphetamines
spices, 141, 226
starches: amylopectin vs. amylose,
39, 47–48; modified, 119; resistant, 40, 48, 50–51, 57. *See also*
carbohydrates
steel cut oats, 43, 45, 49, 50
steroids, 78
stomach: distention, 33, 67; gastric
emptying, 53, 54, 55, 57, 67–68,
70, 71
strawberry, 54, 114, 123
stretching, 146
sucralose, 90, 91
sugar, 39, 199. *See also* blood glucose; carbohydrates; sweeteners,
artificial
Sugar Association, 128
supernormal stimuli, 122–24
surgery, weight-loss (bariatric),
64–65, 71, 79, 174
sweeteners, artificial, 90–91, 119, 123,
131–32
sympathetic tone (sympathetic
nervous system), 33, 35, 72–74,
88, 197

Taleb, Nassim Nicholas, 223, 224
tea, 86, 87–89
testosterone, 33, 74–75, 78

texturizers, 83, 106, 174
theaflavins, 88
thoughts, 200–201. *See also* mindset
"three whys," 20–22
thyroid hormones, 34, 76, 78
tirzepatide (Mounjaro), 71, 79
Torero Cullen, Máximo, 163–64
total energy expenditure (TEE), 18, 19
trans fats, 82–83, 119
Turkey, 8
turmeric, 86, 87
type 1 diabetes, 32
type 2 diabetes, ix–x, 88, 95, 130, 150,
157, 194–95

ultra-processed foods (UPFs): about,
xviii, 100, 102–3; addictiveness,
120, 123–26; avoiding, 116–17,
120, 162–63, 221, 226; Big Tobacco's playbook applied to, 126–29;
Brazil's approach, 99–100, 116;
cheapness, 112–13, 163–64;
common, 118–19; comparison
to satiating foods, 103–4, 106–7,
192–93; convenience, 114; eating
quickly and, 173–74; economic
incentives, 108–9; emotional
eating and, 138–39; as fattening,
107–8; global comparisons, 160;
Golden Rule, 116, 221; "health"
foods as, 226, 227–28; history
of, 109–12; low protein and
fiber, 105; marketing, 115, 134,
164, 221; profitability, 116; real
food mimicry, 113–14; reframing,
203–4; ubiquity of, 161–62; vanishing caloric density, 68, 106;
variety of, 114–15
United Kingdom, 119, 160
United States of America: agricultural subsidies, 163, 164; calories

267

per day compared to obesity
rate, 8; celebratory eating, 177;
misguided dietary advice, 37, 82,
109–11, 193; obesity prevalence,
x, xi, 38, 156; obesogenic environment, 155–58, 159, 161, 164,
214; portion size, 172; protein
consumption, 84–85; ultra-
processed foods consumption,
160
university diet, 147
University of Colorado, 128
University of Toronto, 128

vagus nerve, 33, 67, 145–47
vanishing caloric density, 68, 106
"vegan" milks, 227
vegetables, 58–59, 68, 173, 175, 226,
227
Via Negativa, 224
vinegar, 56
viscosity, food, 55–56
volumetrics, 68

water, sparkling, 90
watermelon, 55
weight gain (obesity): approach to,
xiii–xiv, 230; asking the "three
whys," 21–22; body fat thermostat and, 30–32; correlation to
calories, 8–9; depression and,
139; fattening foods, 14, 35;
hormonal obesity theory, 32–35,
36, 78–79; ignoring the problem, ix–x; insulin and, 14, 16–17,
32, 38, 39, 42, 79, 194; leptin
resistance and, 66; life changes
and, 147–48; menopause and,
75; metabolism and, 41–42;
multifactorial root causes, xvii,
xviii, 7–8, 216–18; obesogenic

environment, 92–93, 155–58,
161–64, 187–88; prevalence, x,
xi, 38, 156; sleep deprivation
and, 69; snacking and, 191–92;
ultra-processed foods and,
107–8
weight loss: approach to, 219–21,
230; automatic weight loss
dietary plan, 224–26, 228–29;
calorie-centric model failure,
x, xv–xvi, 3–4, 4–7, 79, 109–10,
215–16, 219, 223–24; controlling
hunger and satiety, 71; eating
day structure for, 188–90;
Energy Balance Equation and,
9–13; exercise myth, 18–20;
Golden Rules, xv, 221–23; hormones and, 13–17; Lindy Effect
and, 223–24; mindset and, 200;
"not eating" default, 190–91;
sleep and, 69; sympathetic tone
and, 33, 72–74; tips overview,
231–34; Via Negativa and, 224;
willpower myth, 28, 133–34, 136,
155, 191, 215–16. See also fasting;
habits; mindset
weight-loss (bariatric) surgery,
64–65, 71, 79, 174
wheat, 43–44, 48, 163
whey, 57, 85, 105, 113
"whys, three," 20–22
Williams, Vernon B., 145
willpower, 16, 28, 133–34, 136, 155,
187–88, 191, 205, 215–16
Winfrey, Oprah, 215–16
women, 33, 69, 73, 74–75, 147–48
Women's Health Initiative, 5–6

Yale Food Addiction Scale (YFAS), 129
yoga, 146

DID YOU LIKE *THE HUNGER CODE*?
CHECK OUT JASON FUNG'S OTHER BOOKS

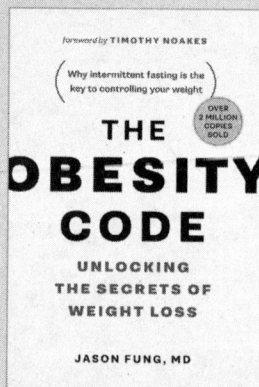

The Obesity Code

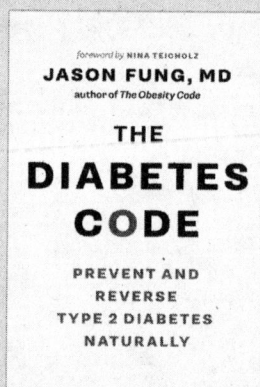

The Diabetes Code

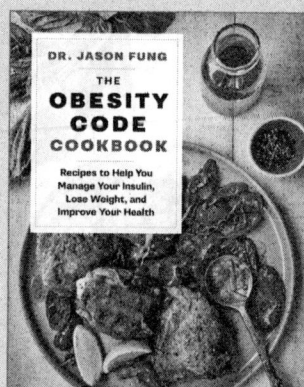

The Obesity Code Cookbook

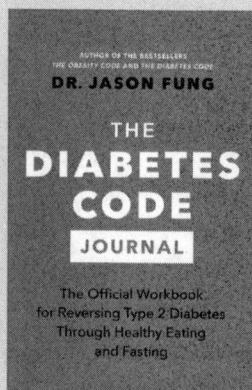

The Diabetes Code Journal

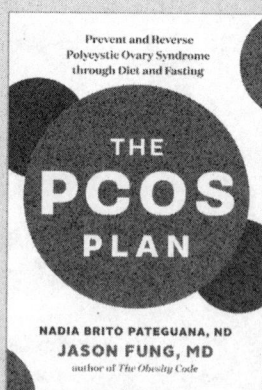

The PCOS Plan

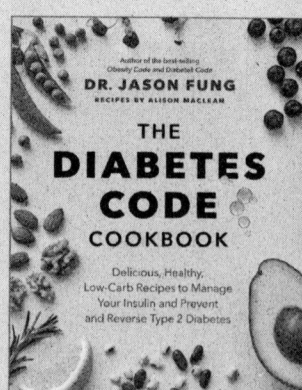

The Diabetes Code Cookbook